Charlotte,
Keep on Smiling!
Ohmedski
Tom

COVID CONVERSATIONS

Voices from Lawrence & Lowell, Massachusetts

COVID CONVERSATIONS

Voices from Lawrence & Lowell, Massachusetts

EDITED BY

Susan Grabski, Amita Kiley, and Susan Tripathy

A PARTNERSHIP PROJECT OF

Lawrence History Center and UMass Lowell,
with contributions from Phillips Academy Andover

ℙ

Loom Press
Amesbury, Massachusetts
2023

To all who lived through the Covid-19 pandemic
and in memory of those we lost.

Contents

Acknowledgements

This book represents the contributions of many people in the greater Lowell and Lawrence communities. First and foremost, we would like to thank everyone who shared their pandemic stories with us and gave permission for them to be included in this book. In Lowell, this includes Sreivuthy Hak, Anábriela Surillo-Navarro, William Chan, Jessica Wilson, Felicia Sullivan, Xavier Robbins, and Miranda Melo. In Lawrence, we are grateful to Vilma Martínez-Dominguez, Carina Pappalardo, Sara Morin Barth, Tom Coppinger, Cristie Galíndez, Dr. Marianela Rivera and Bianca Anonas. We would also like to thank the students at UMass Lowell who conducted the Lowell interviews: Jenna Solomine, Nejaray Torres, Amir Cedeno, Jonathan Hohler, Rebecca Phillips, SreyNich Song, and Samantha DeMonico, and the students at Phillips Academy who conducted the Lawrence interviews: Melani G., Emilia S., Saffron A., Lily R., Gloria C., Carly P., Diego E., Amelia V., Henry C., Bryan J., and Laura O. In addition to overseeing his students' work, we are grateful to Phillips Academy Spanish language instructor Mark Cutler for conducting one of the Lawrence interviews. We would also like to thank Amanda O., Marlin M., Hannah G., Laura C., Jessica M., Hannah V., Jack B., Ryan R., Zariel O., and David G., whose Lawrence Community Diary entries you can read. Clearly, without the generosity and enthusiasm of everyone who agreed to be interviewed or submit a diary entry, as well as those who conducted the interviews, collecting and preserving these experiences during the Covid-19 pandemic would never have been possible.

Once the stories were collected, the work of transcribing, editing, and designing the book began. For this, we would like to acknowledge the contribution of Nejaray Torres, an English major and recent alum of UMass Lowell who completed the initial editing of the Lowell interviews. Christopher Medeiros and Cameron DaCosta are also students at UMass Lowell who assisted with this book: Christopher transcribed, proofread, and edited several Lawrence interviews, and Cameron contributed to the beginning stages of the book design. Lawrence History Center volunteer Kirstin Clarke, Middlesex Community College intern William Heath, and Phillips Academy students Diego E., Gloria C., Carly P., Saffron A., and Lily R. helped with the interview transcriptions. We are also grateful to UMass Lowell student Ashley Rosario for completing the book design, including the artwork on the cover. Her work on the cover was supported by a Future Leaders grant received by Lawrence History Center from the Essex National Heritage Area. In Lowell, thanks are due to Elizabeth Pellerito for encouraging us to collect these interviews in the first place and connecting us with potential interviewees. Tooch Van also helped greatly by sharing information about our project within his social network, and Mee Xiong provided very useful advice about community outreach. We would also like to acknowledge Anthony Sampas at the UMass Lowell Center for Lowell History for providing crucial assistance with consent forms and agreeing to archive the Lowell interviews.

Finally, we are indebted to UMass Lowell College of Fine Arts, Humanities, and Social Sciences Dean Luis Falcón for his generous financial support, and to UMass Lowell History Professor Robert Forrant for encouraging us to create this book. Our commitment to publishing oral histories drew inspiration from *The Big Move: Immigrant Voices from a Mill City*, which was co-authored by Forrant and UMass Lowell History Professor Christoph Strobel. We also thank Robert Forrant for connecting us with Paul Marion and John Wooding at Loom Press, both of whom provided invaluable editorial assistance and support for this project.

Susan Grabski, Lawrence History Center
Amita Kiley, Lawrence History Center
Susan Tripathy, University of Massachusetts Lowell

A Note on Transcription

The interviews presented in this book have been transcribed and edited in a multi-stage process. First, they were transcribed directly from the recordings via transcription software or by one of the people who helped us with transcriptions. If transcription software was used, the transcript was double-checked for accuracy and any necessary corrections were made. Copies of the Lowell transcripts are archived at the Center for Lowell History (https://libguides.uml.edu/archives) and the Lawrence interviews are archived at the Lawrence History Center (www.lawrencehistory.org).

After the initial transcription, the transcripts were edited for clarity and readability, taking care to preserve the unique voice of each interviewee. In some cases, sections of the original interviews were deleted to avoid repetition and focus more directly on experiences during the Covid-19 pandemic. All of the interviewees were provided a copy of their interview to read and approve before publication.

Introduction

Historically, pandemics have forced humans to break with the past and imagine their world anew. This one is no different. It is a portal, a gateway between one world and the next.
—Arundhati Roy (*Financial Times*, April 3, 2020)

March 2020. In Lowell, students went off for spring break thinking they might return in a few weeks. In Lawrence, the schools and local businesses were closed for two weeks, which then led to months. The Covid-19 pandemic disrupted our lives suddenly and with enduring effects. Life changed worldwide and in our own local communities, affecting all our institutions: schools, hospitals, nursing homes, shelters, grocery stores, restaurants, transportation systems, and families. Simultaneously, faults in our social system—racism, classism, and sexism—exacerbated an unequal burden of disease. How did people from a variety of backgrounds cope with this situation? What were their experiences and fears, and how did they get assistance if needed? What, if anything, was positive about the pandemic? And what was being done by community leaders, non-profits, and city, state, and national governments to provide support?

To document this profound period of suffering, loss, sacrifice, adjustment, creativity, and change, this book provides oral histories collected from people living and/or working in Lowell, Mass. or Lawrence, Mass. during the first year of the pandemic. In Lowell, the interviews were conducted by students at UMass Lowell, and in Lawrence, by students from Phillips Academy Andover associated with the Lawrence History Center (LHC). Preserving these stories and making them public builds our collective memory of the Covid-19 pandemic, revealing individual experiences and community perspectives that otherwise might be forgotten. While some aspects of the first year of the pandemic were common for everyone: lockdown, mask-wearing, quarantines, etc., it is through the details of individual stories that you can see the incredible variety of life during this time. These diverse personal pathways through the first year of the pandemic may also provide insights to help prepare for the next pandemic—and in years to come, document how individuals and communities faced new challenges as the coronavirus took hold. As Vilma Martínez-Dominguez, Community Development Director for the City of Lawrence, commented: "Life is not going to be the same again. How do we incorporate the voices of everyone, particularly those who are most vulnerable?"

Lowell and Lawrence, Massachusetts: Inextricably linked

In the early 1800s, a group of wealthy merchants turned industrialists known as the "Boston Associates" developed the city of Lowell as one of the first planned industrial cities. Their investment in Lowell kicked off the American Industrial Revolution. They soon sought to replicate the success they found in Lowell. The Merrimack River and its natural falls proved invaluable as a source of power and cut through plenty of undeveloped land both up and downstream from Lowell.

Just ten miles downriver from the burgeoning textile center of Lowell were the rural towns of Methuen and Andover and the meeting of the Merrimack, Shawsheen, and Spicket Rivers. The Boston Associates chartered a holding company in 1845 called the Essex Company to purchase roughly seven square miles of family-owned farmland in Andover and Methuen. Next, the Essex Company planned the construction of a dam to provide the waterpower necessary for the mills they envisioned lining the river. The Great Stone Dam as it became known created the foundation for the future growth of the city of Lawrence.

The directors of the Essex Company included the interlocked families—the Lawrences, Lowells, Appletons, Jacksons, and many others—who controlled most of the New England textile industry and were influential in the early development of the railroad in New England. They were also largely responsible for the growth of the major institutions and cityscape of nearby Boston. Since the mid-19th century, both Lowell and Lawrence have served as gateway cities for immigrants and refugees arriving and settling in the United States.

How our project started

Before coming together to create this book, this oral history project had two beginnings: one in Lowell and one in Lawrence. In Lowell, during the summer of 2020, Susan Tripathy was preparing to teach Sociology of Health and Healthcare via Zoom during the Fall semester at UMass Lowell and was looking for a project that could be done virtually but still allow students to connect with people in the community. Very soon after the start of the pandemic, a new mutual assistance organization had been formed in Lowell—LLAMA, Lifting Lowellians: Assistance and Mutual Aid. After a conversation with one of the founders of this organization, UMass Lowell Labor Education Program Director Elizabeth Pellerito, Susan decided that engaging her class in an oral history project, with the goal of listening and learning from people who lived, worked, or attended school in Lowell, would provide valuable historical documentation as well as contemporary insight into how the Lowell community was affected by the pandemic. When she introduced this project to her class of twenty-three students, they were enthusiastic, and so "The Pandemic Story Project" was born.

To prepare for the interviews, the class learned oral history techniques and also heard presentations by Elizabeth Pellerito about LLAMA and UMass Lowell History Professor Robert Forrant about the history of Lowell, in particular background on different immigrant/refugee groups in the city. Susan also reached out to Anthony Sampas at the UMass Lowell Center for Lowell History, who agreed to archive the interviews and helped finalize consent forms. Following the advice of Mee Xiong from UMass

Lowell's Southeast Asian Digital Archive (SEADA), she then set up a website via Google sites to advertise the project and connect with people who were willing/interested to share their stories. Considering the wide range of languages spoken in Lowell, the class decided offering a variety of languages would be important. The students themselves had proficiency in Spanish, Khmer, Vietnamese, French, and English. So on the website, we mentioned that people could choose to have their interviews in any of these languages. However, all of our interviewees for this collection chose to be interviewed in English.

Nejaray Torres, a student in this class, is an English major who has previously conducted interviews and written for regional publications. In addition to completing her own interview, after the class was finished she provided editorial support for this project and then continued in this capacity after she graduated with her bachelor's degree in May 2021. For Nejaray, interviewing a UMass Lowell student (who was not in the course) about her everyday life during the pandemic was an enlightening experience. She was able to see how another person, who was very similar to herself, was coping with Covid-19. You can read the interview she conducted with Anábriela Surillo-Navarro in this book (page 90). Through the editing of her classmates' interviews, Nejaray understood that during this chaotic time, many people were having some of the same experiences but in different ways. It reminded her of the theme of unity through a lonely time. The Covid-19 pandemic called for people to isolate themselves from family members and loved ones, and the virus changed many aspects of day-to-day life for those interviewed.

All students in the class completed at least one interview, and a few did two interviews, for a total of twenty-five finished interviews. Depending on the preference of the interviewee, some of the interviews were completed via Zoom and others over the telephone. Each student was responsible for transcribing the interview(s) they conducted. All of these interviews have been archived at the Center for Lowell History.

Turning to Lawrence, the Lawrence History Center had a long-standing oral history program in place when the pandemic shut down the city in mid-March 2020. The organization began conducting oral histories in 1978, the year of its founding, using tape recorders. Its oral history collection includes approximately 700 audio tapes that have been digitally mastered, some with eyewitness accounts going as far back as the 1912 Lawrence Textile Strike (also known as the Bread and Roses Strike). Interviews cover a variety of subjects (e.g., military services, immigration, schools, churches, neighborhoods, labor, clubs & organizations, social services, family and civic life, and urban renewal).

As digital technologies emerged, some of the early volunteers and staff who conducted the interviews retired. In an effort to continue capturing individual stories, LHC expanded its efforts to obtain oral and video histories through community partnerships. For example, in 2012 the blog "We, the People: Voices of the Immigrant City" (http://www.lawrencehistory.org/collections/oralhistories/wethepeople) was created by Phillips Academy Spanish language instructor Mark Cutler (now the president of the LHC Board of Directors) and his students. The collection of video oral history interviews is the result of a complex but vibrant collaboration between youths and adults committed to community development and to the idea that one, single story does not define a place. And the interviews are now a part of the LHC archival collections.

In mid-March 2020, the scheduling of spring interviews was already in motion. Interviews were to be conducted in the traditional in-person manner. When the world shut down, LHC saw this moment in time as an opportunity to capture the stories of our community members and leaders in real time. In turn, in early April 2020, we transitioned our traditional oral history program to virtual by launching the bilingual project, "Remote Oral History: Physically Distanced. Socially Connected" (www.

lawrencehistory.org/collections/remoteoralhistory).

The transition required that all interviews be conducted virtually on Zoom. And it also included moving paper forms, e.g., oral history agreement forms, permissions, and terms and conditions, to an online form powered by Jotform that allowed us to capture signatures in a secure way. Because of the changes to the process, we developed what we called a "primer" or best practices document to guide our efforts. The primer includes information about what remote oral history is, what its limitations are, how one goes about capturing oral histories remotely (invitation, pitch, setting up and recording the interview), transcription, permissions, and overall guidance on the process and eventual donation of interview to the LHC archival collection (see page 177).

As spring of 2020 progressed, LHC, along with Mark Cutler and his Spanish language course students, captured stories of the community coming together in times of crisis. Seven full-length interviews were conducted with people in city government, heads of human service organizations (addressing homelessness, substance use, mental illness), teachers, community gardeners, and members of the LHC board and community. As we moved into 2021 an additional five interviews were conducted.

Also in 2020, we launched the bilingual Lawrence Community Diary. We were inspired by the diaries of a young woman, Helen Annie Benker, written in 1918 and 1920 during the influenza pandemic and held in the LHC collection. We invited our community to make a diary entry (or daily entries!) about their experience living in Lawrence during the 2020 Covid-19 pandemic at www.lawrencehistory.org/collections/remoteoralhistory/diary. We received dozens of entries, and that number continues to grow as local teachers incorporated the diary project into their classroom assignments. Entries have ranged from expressions of boredom with the Netflix offerings after being home for so long to apprehension about attending outdoor public gatherings in the wake of the death of George Floyd to heartbreaking entries like one from a young person who lost his father in the Dominican Republic, but was unable to travel to be there with him prior to his passing. We have included ten in this book from students, professionals, and community members ranging in age from fourteen to fifty-five. Later, to ensure equality of access, we also added a bilingual Google voice number for those not wanting to submit their thoughts in writing and/or to be video-taped.

The project garnered attention from the Essex National Heritage Area, the Essex County Community Foundation, the Phillips Library of the Peabody Essex Museum, the Massachusetts History Alliance, and the New England Archivists. Ellan Spero, a professor at Massachusetts Institute of Technology who was key to establishing Station1 in Lawrence (www.station1.org/) and with whom we've worked on building humanities-based STEM curriculum, shared the project with the Leonardi DaVinci National Science and Technology Museum in Milan, Italy, as an example of how to engage new audiences.

When Susan Grabski, Executive Director of the Lawrence History Center, learned about this book project, the need to have the interviews transcribed quickly was clear. Using video transcriptions generated by YouTube, in tandem with careful repeat reviews of the video recordings, several individuals from Phillips Academy, UMass Lowell, Middlesex Community College, and Lawrence History Center did this work. Amita Kiley, Collections Manager and Research Coordinator at LHC, supervised the transcription work and also edited the transcripts.

How we selected the oral histories included in this book

While each interview tells a unique story and choosing between them was difficult, we selected interviews we felt illustrated diverse experiences people dealt with—both positive and negative. We wanted to represent voices from a variety of socio-economic classes, ethnic/racial groups, and ages, as well as from people working in different types of local businesses and organizations. As we continued to read over the interviews, we decided to group them according to main themes: Learning, Teaching, and Studying; Providing Healthcare: Rehabilitation Centers and Nursing Homes; Family, Work, and Community; and Community Organizations and Mutual Aid. In the Learning, Teaching, and Studying section, you can read about Sreivuthy Hak's experience returning to her family's home in Cambodia and continuing to take classes via Zoom at UMass Lowell. Bianca Anonas, a U.S. History teacher at Lawrence High School who was born in Manila, Philippines, speaks about how she has dealt with the challenges of the pandemic in order to keep teaching and helping her students. Cristie Galíndez describes the challenges of teaching five- and six-year-olds basic school skills such as how to hold a pencil over Zoom. And Dr. Marianela Rivera tells the story of her struggles against racial inequality and inequity, and the adversity she faced in her academic career. Under Providing Healthcare, you'll hear about Miranda Melo's responsibilities as a new nursing graduate managing Covid testing at a nursing home, and Xavier Robbins' work at a rehabilitation center in addition to his amazing new business customizing shoes. Tom Coppinger, the director of the Point After Club in Lawrence, speaks about how this provider of rehabilitation services to people with mental illnesses continued to serve its members remotely. Turning to Family, Work, and Community, Jessica Wilson provides an up-front view of directing a nonprofit, Mill City Grows, while simultaneously parenting a young child. Anábriela Surillo-Navarro describes a trip to visit her family in Puerto Rico, and in William Chan's interview, a dialogue develops with the interviewer, Jonathan Hohler, which leads to a comparison of pandemic life in a mostly Cambodian neighborhood in Lowell with that of a White, economically advantaged neighborhood in Reading. Sara Morin, born in Guatemala City, Guatemala before being adopted and emigrating to Methuen,

Massachusetts, shares stories of the Lawrence community's resiliency through her work at the Greater Lawrence Community Action Council as well as of her deep family ties to her grandmother, now in a nursing home, and the emotional difficulties of having to postpone her wedding to a date then unknown. Finally, in Community Organizations and Mutual Aid, Felicia Sullivan takes us back to the first few months of the pandemic to describe how LLAMA (Lifting Lowellians: Assistance and Mutual Aid) was started. Carina Pappalardo, Chief Executive Officer for The Psychological Center in Lawrence, Mass., speaks about never giving up on her efforts to protect and ensure respect and dignity to those affected by mental health challenges, addiction and/or homelessness despite the barriers imposed by the public health crisis. Vilma Martínez-Dominguez, Community Development Director for the City of Lawrence and co-founder of the Mayor's Health Task Force (born of her decades-long work for the YWCA) emphasizes the importance of civic responsibility, partnerships, and empowering the citizens of Lawrence during and after the pandemic.

As the Pandemic Continued . . .

As of June 2022, efforts are underway at both the Lawrence History Center and UMass Lowell to expand on this collection of oral histories of the Covid-19 pandemic. In Lawrence, the oral history program continued during Spring Semester 2021 with an additional seven interviews, and more are planned through 2022. At UMass Lowell, Sokharath Koy, an honors sociology major, interviewed six members of Lowell's Cambodian community in Khmer for his senior honors project. These interviews were transcribed in both Khmer and English. During spring 2022, we also recontacted all the people interviewed for this book and asked how their lives had changed since their initial interview in 2020. You can read these updates in a paragraph immediately following each interview.

We hope that you will enjoy the stories told by members of the Greater Lowell and Greater Lawrence communities—captured in different places, from different perspectives—during the first year of the Covid-19 pandemic. Gathering, preserving, and interpreting the voices and memories of people, communities, and participants in past events is the oldest type of historical inquiry, predating the written word. Doing so not only helps us to document the past, but to learn from it as we move into the future.

Prologue

We invited Dr. Gregory R. Chiklis and Dr. Demetrius P. Rizos, both alumni of UMass Lowell, to share their observations and experiences in the early days of the Covid-19 pandemic. Their frontline work was part of the vast health care and research efforts in the U.S. and around the world. Their accounts provide further context for the stories of people in this book whose lives were dramatically altered by the virus. The vivid oral histories spell out the daily challenges and responses that are now part of the regional record of the crisis.

I remember this as if it was yesterday. In 2002, I received a call from the Centers for Disease Control and Prevention (CDC) Respiratory Division head to assist their quality control team with a new severe acute respiratory syndrome (SARS) polymerase chain reaction (PCR) test. The SARS outbreak had started in China and, through a research collaboration, the CDC already had the viral sequence and were growing it in culture. With these variables in place, it didn't take long for the CDC to develop diagnostic test kits and components to track the spread of the virus. Test availability allowed us to quickly identify infected individuals, isolate them from the general population, and stop its spread. Ultimately, approximately eight thousand people were infected with an eleven percent fatality rate. Since 2004, there have been no new cases. The virus was defeated.

At the beginning of this current pandemic, I remember watching the news about this new strain of severe acute respiratory syndrome coronavirus 2 (SARS CoV-2) virus and how the Chinese government started to lock down major cities with populations greater than twenty-five million. We had no viral diagnostic or sequence information because the Chinese government would not share information. It became obvious to me that it was just a matter of time before it spread globally. A month later after the Chinese New Year celebrations, passengers traveled from Wuhan on planes spreading the infection to countries all over the world.

Unfortunately, we had to wait for the virus to come to the U.S. before it could be isolated and sequenced. The delay in test development cost hundreds of thousands of lives globally. Because we had no way to detect the virus, the U.S. Food and Drug Administration (FDA) issued an Emergency Use Act, which allowed for minimal data requirements to get tests onto the market. It also allowed many international tests with only limited development data to enter the market as well. This was a recipe for disaster, as unreliable tests caused both confusion and false positive diagnoses.

To support diagnostic test researchers, we pivoted our company to focus only on Covid diagnostics. We worked as quickly as possible with our diagnostic clients to validate accurate tests while working to fix inaccurate tests currently in the market. We created drive-up carports for swab collections, which we used to provide samples for diagnostic test development and FDA test kit submissions. We also provided some of these samples to UMass Lowell Professor Matthew Gage who, with his team, developed a saliva pool test for the university. This was amazing work by Dr. Gage and his group and was done at a time when everyone else was locked down. This testing and identification and isolation of infected students was a large factor in the low outbreak levels that were seen at the University. Needless to say it was a constant race against a rapidly spreading virus and we worked diligently to develop as many accurate tests as possible.

At our Florida blood banks, we also pivoted from collecting normal whole blood to therapeutic plasma—called CCP (convalescent plasma). This is collected from a Covid recovered donor and contains high concentrations of Covid antibodies to treat sick individuals. Finally, to ensure end users were running the tests correctly, we developed Covid proficiency testing panels and sent them to 3500 domestic laboratories to make sure they understood how to run the tests. Finally, we carried out many untrained user validation studies to help develop simple home kits for those without a health care provider. Today, these tests are readily available in commercial pharmacies as over-the-counter tests.

Although the pandemic has adversely affected us, it was a time to unite families during lockdown. Also, the scientific community reached levels of collaboration that I have never seen in my career. Throughout the pandemic, we were supported by research scientists, the federal government, other diagnostic companies, U.S. blood donors, local community leaders, and benevolent residents who provided clinical testing samples for our development and validation studies. We are prepared for the future, as we now have many new tools for development of these rapid diagnostic tests. This transformation to rapid easy-to-use home tests or pharmacy testing, is a tremendously positive shift in our industry, as it allows access of diagnostic tests for everyone. Today we are developing combination rapid assays for these point of care sites for viruses like influenza A/B, respiratory syncytial virus (RSV), Covid, and others. These positive testing advancements were the direct result of this pandemic and will benefit everyone through easy access to future diagnostic tests.

Gregory R. Chiklis, Ph.D.
Chief Executive Officer
MRN Diagnostics
University of Massachusetts Lowell, '92

From April through June of 2020, I had the privilege to treat critically ill Covid-19 patients in the Bronx. I've never been on a battlefield, but it was very much like being on the front lines of a medical disaster.

Although my colleagues & I lacked access to both preventative and therapeutic anti-viral therapies, we had a collaborative *esprit de corps* and worked tirelessly to keep a great number of patients safe from harm's way.

This very same collaborative spirit has embodied the Massachusetts sister cities of Lowell and Lawrence for over 150 years. Immigrants worked tirelessly to establish communities, build churches, work in mills, and raise families. They may have been poor, but they were both rich in determination and thankful for what little they had.

It does not surprise anyone that, during the past twenty-four plus months, these communities exhibited this same resolve. Ill patients were both protected and treated, education was propagated, complicated university research was performed at warp speed, and community bonds were fortified.

The Greek philosopher Epictetus stated, "It's not what happens to you, but how you react to it that matters." This is more than exemplified by the Merrimack Valley's ongoing fortitude and community spirit.

Demetrius P. Rizos, DO, FACP, FASN
LCDR, MC, USNR
Brigham & Women's Hospital
University of Lowell, '91

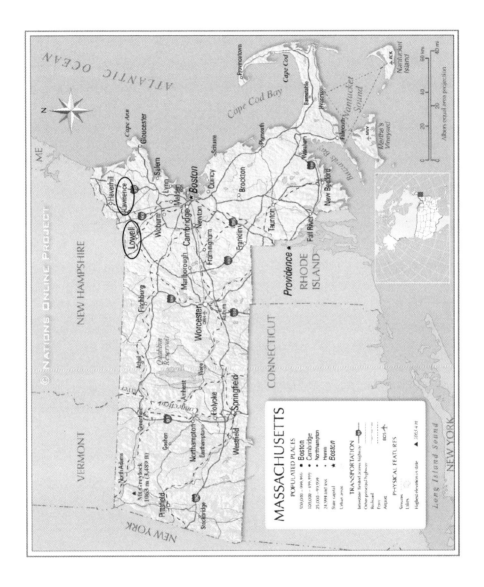

Used with permission from the Nations Online Project
https://www.nationsonline.org/oneworld/map/USA/massachusetts_map.htm

I.

Learning, Teaching, and Studying

Bianca Anonas
Lawrence High School U.S. History teacher

Sreivuthy Hak
UMass Lowell student

Dr. Marianela Rivera
*Advocate and Activist for Educational Activism, Public Education
Organizer for Massachusetts Jobs for Justice, physical therapist*

Cristie Galíndez
Teacher at the John Breen School in Lawrence

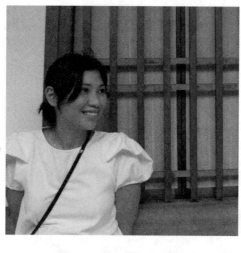

Bianca Anonas

"I was telling my kids that what you're living in is historical. This is what it might have felt like to be in America when there was rationing in World War II."

Bianca Anonas is a thirty-five-year-old U.S. History teacher and moderator for the Charity Club at Lawrence High School. She was born in Manila, Philippines, and immigrated to the United States. She speaks about how she has dealt with the challenges of the pandemic to keep teaching and helping her students.

Bianca was interviewed by Phillips Academy students Melani G. and Emilia S. on May 5, 2020.

My name is Bianca Anonas; I am a teacher at Lawrence High School. I am actually an immigrant. I came here from Manila, Philippines, in, I want to say, officially 2010, so I've been living in the Chelmsford/Lowell area ever since.

We can get started by talking about what you do, what your job is, and your association with Lawrence.

I wear different hats in Lawrence in a sense, but I'm a history teacher, primarily. I teach U.S. History II, and I'm also a OneGoal teacher, which is basically helping students with their post-secondary careers, whether it's college, community college, or tech school, especially students who might be high-risk. And the other thing is this year I'm the moderator of the Charity Club at Lawrence High School. I think that's about it.

What's your home situation like—who are you living with?

I live with my family, family meaning my husband and my four-year-old son. Since I moved here, I don't really have family in the area, and my husband is originally from Pennsylvania so it's kind of just us self-isolating, quarantining, social distancing.

You talked about how you were staying with your family right now social distancing and quarantining. Do you think that being an immigrant makes this easier?

I think if I were to talk about my husband's experience, he wants to visit his parents, but he doesn't think it's safe. He wants to be able to see them at some point. But as for me, the social distancing isn't a problem because I haven't seen my parents in over two years, or three years. We were supposed to go back this summer which is probably not happening. So, in a sense the social distancing is easy, but as an immigrant we have all these plans. My brother is getting married this coming summer so you had all these plans, and things you were looking forward to, but now it's very disappointing.

How do you think Lawrence High is managing the pandemic, and what do you think it has lost due to this pandemic?

I think I'll focus on the positive stuff first. Teachers have really come together to help each other out, but also to reach out to their students. I know teachers are finding so many different ways to reach out to their students, even if it's calling them from home, emailing them, downloading remind apps, Google class-room and all of these things, to make sure that they're just okay. We have some students who are really good who probably will finish with an A, but we've heard zero from them, so it's like are they okay? I think in terms of the bigger picture, Lawrence Public Schools has been really good with dispersing electronic devices or technology to the students, considering that it's a district of over 13,000 students. I know they've given at least one laptop per family. Plus they are also providing students with internet access for those who don't have any, so it's really just trying to move as quickly as possible given the limitations. One thing that I feel we're also navigating right now is some students are doing well online, not saying that everybody is, but there's still some quality work that we're receiving, and students are also adapting themselves to work online.

Something that we've lost. I feel like Lawrence is an immigrant city and thinking about all our ELL or English Language Learners, they don't get exposure to the English language outside of school. I think we're going to see real discrepancies and language issues when we come back. So, on top of the subject matter, the content, those skills, there's also that language thing that's worrisome. A lot of our kids are also working more during this time, which worries the teachers, and I'm sure worries their families. But it's also not just their students, but their families working a lot and trying to figure out some day-to-day things like loss of income and stuff like that.

You were mentioning about how students don't have that much exposure outside of school to talk in English. Is the school changing the curriculum next year to accommodate what Covid-19 has caused?

Lawrence has ESL classes. So on top of your English, math, science, the content, those who are marked as English Language Learners have those additional support classes. But if you've listened to anything like the news and the Department of Elementary and Secondary Education in the state, it's not just Lawrence, but it's the whole state that has to rework some of these skills that might be lost or there might be a deficit in those specific skills. Because technically if a student hasn't done any work during this time or hasn't done any school, it's almost like SLIFE (Students with Limited or Interrupted Formal Education), where it's interrupted learning, so we're hoping that there will be some support when we come back. But at the same time, we don't know. I guess from a teacher's perspective we hope there is, but that might be more for administration to figure out or maybe the English as a Second Language Department.

Since all these things have been happening, how has your teaching in particular changed?

This is my third year in LHS. I originally was a teacher, but in an untraditional hospital setting, and I really wanted to come back to more of a traditional classroom and in a district with diversity. I applied to one or two districts just to see what happened. I've been with Lawrence for three years now and I love working here, I love the kids, I like the people that I work with, so it's been really good. In terms of adapting my teaching in this particular time, I am trying to learn, I guess, ways to communicate, not just Zoom, but even like Flipgrid. I have two classes that are fifty percent or something like that, or maybe a little less than fifty percent ELLs. So I have a co-teacher there, but even thinking about how if I put a reading up I'm going to supplement that with recording myself reading the reading. Or recording myself going over a PowerPoint that they might not be able to do just by themselves or something that might be difficult for them to understand. Also chunking lessons into smaller increments so it's not overwhelming. I can't put a five-page something for them to read and do, I split it up like part one, part two, just to make it better, especially for those who might be struggling with a lot of long or heavy material.

Can you talk a little bit about why you got into teaching in the first place?

I think it's because I always loved school. A lot of my friends now are people who I've worked with. Since I've had good relationships with my teachers, I guess I'm the type of student who they would be in touch with even if I've graduated. I heard this piece of advice: If you want to be a teacher, hang out with teachers and see how that is, and they were my people, I guess. So it's that love for learning plus my love for being able to share things that I find really important or interesting to other people.

Going back to how you've had to change some things around in your teaching, is there anything that remote learning is teaching you? And is there anything you're hoping to carry back into the classroom once this all blows over?

With remote learning you can see certain students are doing better because maybe they're more introverted compared to when they are in the classroom. So what it's teaching me, is that we really need to incorporate remote learning in the classroom with face-to-face. Just because there are limitations, as well, there's only X amount of laptop cards for this amount of population. I'm really hoping that every student will be able to have a laptop so that remote learning can be taught at the very beginning of a school year, and it becomes something that they can get more used to. Because we're finding that compared to other districts where they've had the laptop at the beginning or even like other classes where it's computer-based work, the kids are having no issues doing the work versus this is something new. So really having that balance—hopefully we get to do more face-to-face. Other things, too. I like the new technology that I've learned. Flipgrid is one that I want to be able to use. And even using Google Classroom a little bit more in my classes than just once a month. Before the pandemic I would probably use it five times. I'm making it more regular to get kids used to it because I feel like that's also how it's going to be more useful for them if they go to college.

We wanted to talk to you about before quarantine and how the teaching space was in the classroom. I know that in your audio you mentioned your experiences being an Asian or Asian American teacher in the classroom.

My experience was you could hear more kids mentioning it in front of me or asking me about what I know about the virus. I asked my other history teachers, "Are you guys getting as many questions about Covid-19 as I am?" And they said, "No, not really." I wondered why that was. So I feel like it's kind of a mix of students who think they are being funny, acting immature, but also it's a good opportunity to open up discussion. To be able to ask, "Why are you asking me that question if I'm not a doctor?" Or even in talking about my Asian heritage, which isn't Chinese, and letting them learn to be more sensitive in how they approach it. Being more open about that and making it a learning opportunity. But there are also some students who will be like "Miss, that's messed up." The students like to call out one another like, "That's not cool." So that's a good thing that other students are sensitive to, and they can pick that up and call each other out. It is different, too, when a teacher calls out a student than when a student is calling another student out. It has a different impact. I think that is interesting. I didn't really experience hurtful, scary racism, unlike the articles you've read in different parts of the country, like in New York. I feel like it was just more immaturity, but also a lack of knowledge and understanding. Lawrence has a more Hispanic population, I want to say eighty percent or more are Spanish. So even thinking about how on the national level where you have Donald Trump saying all Mexicans are rapists, drug dealers, etc., that negative view of the Hispanic community shifts in these times to another minority group. It's almost like, Thank God it's not us that they're putting in the spotlight. You know the crisis can bring the worst and the best.

How does that make you feel?

It makes me nervous. I'm kind of like, Oh my God, I'm glad I'm in Massachusetts, not somewhere else because even when I cross the border to New Hampshire I feel like there is some sketchy racism going on. I think it makes me feel like I need to be more vigilant, personally, and more safe, especially when I'm with my four-year-old. And sometimes I have to think, What if this happened, how would I react? If it happened to you on the spot you want to be able to keep yourself safe and also still be able to engage in a more positive way so that it doesn't become angry shouting or anything. I think that's where my frame of mind is, like well if this happened maybe I could do this, or if this happened would I even engage or just walk away. There are a lot of positive things because there are people who will stand up for you. But again as a history teacher, this isn't anything new unfortunately. Right now, what I did with a lesson is I juxtaposed the Japanese-American internment camps because we were finishing up World War II, versus the experience of Asian Americans today. So even having students think about looking at this part in history versus today—What are things that you can do as a positive? As a responsible citizen? Making them think about those things that make them aware historically isn't new, but at the same time we have to be able to make certain choices or do things that are more positive and be more upstanders, be more aware if this is happening.

I'm assuming that you've seen your students' writing in the LHC community diary—what kind of reflections are you having from that?

I did a quick reflection activity before the LHC had theirs, so I was already reading some stuff from the students and there were key reflections that may be/can be shared. I had prompts, which is why it's very specific. A lot of them do miss school. They first were really pumped that school was going to be cancelled, but I don't think they realized the impact of that and how long it was going to be. So maybe there's a new appreciation for school and for being there for teachers. A lot of the kids are working more in Market Basket or Dunkin', those places that are open, but also, I guess some of them are trying to keep safe at the same time, there are others around them that aren't. There was one student who mentioned that she's not even Hispanic and she feels that there is still racism in general towards immigrants. Basically, not because Asian Americans are quote-unquote "being the problem" but just immigrants in general, because she expressed that she experienced some racism while going to the food store.

Do you think you can talk a little bit more about your immigrant experience?

I came here to study, to get an education degree. I went to Tufts University in 2008 for grad school, and I met my husband there. After two years, we decided to get married, and he preferred to stay here. I officially moved here in 2010. The thing with my immigrant experience that's a little bit different than others is that I know how to speak English, so it wasn't too too much of a change in terms of communication, even culturally, because the Philippines was under American control after 1898 and I mean strongly influenced up until the 1940s and '50s, and still strongly influenced indirectly today. Being exposed to the language really helped me assimilate. But still many cultural differences, like going to a supermarket—those big Stop & Shops scared me. There's so much food here! There's like Google aisles of ice cream where in the Philippines it's one freezer! Even seeing people . . . because some parts of Asia are more homogeneous, but even being with different people, different races, ethnicities, it was like a mind shift almost and especially at Tufts where predominantly it's White, so almost feeling like I'm in another world. Those little things that make you realize that you're not home, but at the same time like now, I feel like I'm part of both worlds. It's weird because as an immigrant you feel like you're part of both worlds, but at the same time you're not part of both worlds, you're not completely part of both worlds—does that make sense— it's like you're caught in the middle.

My mom says that once you live in more than one place there's no longer a perfect place. She too is an immigrant. Do you think that applies to you, do you agree with that statement?

Yes, there's no perfect place, but also when you go back to your country you see all these changes like that restaurant is no longer there, or oh this is here now. But at the same time it's not necessarily the surroundings that change, but it's you've changed, too, so it's weird. It's also the concept of home, like when people ask you where you are from—and that's a good question. Your concept of home is more like people rather than places, kind of. And if you live in more than one place, I feel like you feel more like a citizen of the world rather than tied down to a specific place. You're like a new culture in yourself or something.

Why did you think to turn to the LHC to tell your story?

I think I wanted to be able to support LHC. LHC was working with my class before all this. We were going to be doing our final projects in March, and that went on the wayside and I was like, no—because we did so much work building up for it. I've been able to meet and speak to people at LHC, and also in the Lawrence Heritage State Park, but it really just stopped. I wanted to help them in this even if I couldn't get my kids to do their final project. Maybe this could be a way that I can make sure my kids share their experiences, but also I can share my experience.

Does being a history teacher add to the value placed on organizations that preserve histories?

Yes, and I was telling my kids that what you're living in is historical. This is what it might have felt like to be like in America when there was rationing in World War II, and it really is up to them to decide what they want to do with themselves given their situation at this particular time. You know you're gonna work okay, but what else can you do? You're gonna do your schoolwork, you got to make those choices, and it's not going to be easy with everything going on.

How are you able to encourage your students to stay motivated and continue to want to do their work, and how are you encouraging yourself to do that?

That's a good question. I think not just me, but all the teachers have been reaching out. We are supposed to call our advisees every week and remind them to do the work. But also, be able to identify students who are failing or who have not done a single assignment on Google classroom or whatever. We reach out to them individually or out to their teams like their dean or their advisory teacher to encourage them. When I give feedback to assignments on Google classroom I make sure to write a little note like, I'm so glad to hear from you. If it's the first assignment they've done, I might ask, How are you and your family doing? And thank you so much for doing the work, and things like that. In some of my other classes there's a remind app where you can just send messages to the kids on their phone, so even if you sound like a gif, like fun gifs or memes or whatever works. And as for teacher motivation, really working with my colleagues is motivating, and being able to see some of the good responses from students, even if it's just a few students showing responses or giving quality responses, makes me feel like the work that I'm putting up or the work that I'm putting into creating or modifying a lesson is worth it.

Before we wrap this thing up. is there anything that we missed?

I'm sure I forgot something. There's really a lot that this has taught me and sometimes we can't even articulate what that is. I know if we've learned anything in history it eventually becomes okay. With Lawrence it's such a close-knit community that this has been particularly hard for them. You had the Merrimack Valley gas explosion last year and then there were some gas leaks at the beginning of this school year and so many other things. I think the virus has really highlighted the flaws in the systems that we live in. Also, how socioeconomic status plays a role in who gets impacted more versus others. Lawrence is a resilient community and it's going to get through this and everybody's going to get through this. We just need to remember to work together as human beings.

I guess it surprises me how a lot of people are not following the guidelines like social distancing, which is very frustrating. I have a four-year-old who hasn't had a playdate, who hasn't been with his friends, who is missing all these things. And then you see parents having their kids playing with each other or doing things that they're not supposed to. Then you have my four-year-old saying, I want to do that, and I say, You can't—but why are they doing it? So, it's kind of frustrating considering the sacrifices being made by people who are social distancing and quarantining, etc. It's almost like what other people are doing is negating that sacrifice, so it's like all the work we're doing is for nothing. I have a lot of people who are front liners—nurses, doctors, a lot of my friends and family, and I hear my friends. I have a friend in the Philippines who lost both her uncle and aunt. We lost a doctor—a cardiologist who was seeing my grandma. My husband's father who's a pediatrician, his friend, who's a Filipino doctor in New Jersey, passed from Covid. We know people who have lost their lives and I'm like, Why aren't people taking this seriously? So, we've got to work together, everybody needs to work together.

***

Update

I am still teaching in Lawrence High School, and we are full in person. It has been a very challenging school year, but it has been so great to be with the students in school. I've been working on projects here and there, whether it's with an organization like Facing History or with fellow educators in Lawrence fostering culturally responsive pedagogy. I am feeling more hopeful that things will slowly be getting better. I've been fortunate enough to fulfill a dream and have a once-in-a-lifetime experience during the pandemic. One of my favorite international music groups, Bangtan Seonyandan (BTS), was able to have a concert in America and I was able to go. It may not seem like much to many, but out of their millions of fans all over the world (over forty million to be exact) I was able to see them in person—Bianca Anonas

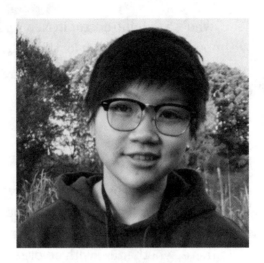

Sreivuthy Hak

"Over here [Cambodia] it's no more different than over there [U.S.] except the time difference. Over here, we're twelve hours ahead. Let's say it's like 1 p.m. over there in the United States, it would be 1 a.m. So, I have to stay up until like 8 p.m. at night all the way to 5 a.m. in the morning to study and to be present at my lectures over here."

Sreivuthy Hak is a twenty-year-old full-time student majoring in business management at UMass Lowell. She identifies as Cambodian-American and has lived in Lowell for ten years. In this interview, Sreivuthy discusses the difficulties of moving back to Cambodia in the middle of a pandemic and simultaneously taking virtual classes at UMass Lowell.

Sreivuthy was interviewed by SreyNich Song on November 14, 2020.

Let's talk about your experiences during the pandemic. How has your life changed during the current Covid-19 pandemic?

Mainly, it changed from me being situated in Lowell, then moving all the way back to my home country in Cambodia.

Is there a particular story you'd like to share about your experience?

The move itself was pretty difficult. I had to give up my room in the apartment, and my stuff had to be put in storage. My car is allocated to my friends to take care of, and my mail as well. So, it was all in a rush, where I had to leave the country as fast as I could to avoid the virus.

Can you explain when you moved and how you made the decision to move?

I moved, I think near the beginning of June or July 2020, somewhere there. It was a really tough decision, because I went back and forth between my parents. My parents, and the rest of my family, wanted me to move there [Cambodia] really fast. And I wanted to stay here because I thought it was fine. Ultimately, they won. So, I had to move all my stuff and basically pack myself in one week. And then all my stuff had to be put in the warehouse within two days, because my flight was already booked. It was a really rushed process.

What is a typical day like for you now?

Over here, it's no more different than over there except the time difference. Over here, we're twelve hours ahead. Let's say it's like 1 p.m. over there in the United States, it would be 1 a.m here. So, I have to stay up until like 8 p.m. at night all the way to 5 a.m. in the morning to study and to be present at my lectures over here.

So, you're still taking classes?

Yeah, I'm currently taking classes.

Why did you make the decision to do that, even though it would be harder on you?

Um, me personally, I have to do what I have to do. And if I take a break for one semester, knowing me, I'll probably forget my lessons and also become lazy to get back into the whole school schedule.

What has been the most challenging for you?

I think the most challenging is the time difference itself because it's not like I'm living alone where I can do whatever I want with my time. I'm living with family. So, if they want to go somewhere, then I have to go with them. During the daytime, if they want to do something, I have to be at work during that time. So, when it comes to the nighttime when I study, I'm really, really sleep deprived.

Has that been taking a toll on your schooling?

Not necessarily. My grades are still doing fine. Um, yeah, I'm just smart.

Has your stress level changed during the pandemic? If so, what do you do to cope with this?

My stress level hasn't really changed, whether I was over there or over here because I typically get to do whatever I want. When it comes to schoolwork and keeping up with the assignments, the business major is pretty easy to handle. So, I don't have anything to complain about academically. I want to say there is not too much stress. The only stress I'm feeling is what am I going to do when I go back? Where am I going to find a place to stay? Or how am I going to move all my stuff back?

Are there any positive aspects to your life during the pandemic?

I get to stay with my family. This is the first time I've stayed with them for more than three months over summer break. So, that's a nice change from living alone.

Do you mainly live alone when you're in Lowell?

Yeah.

How did you receive help, if you needed it?

Well, academically, I don't receive any help. I don't ask for any help. But personally, over here, they accommodate most of my needs. Like, if I'm studying in the middle of the night, then I might need food to hold my stomach. So, my family would make extra food or leave extra food in the fridge. Everyone does a really good job of accommodating my situation. So, I wouldn't say I need to ask for anything much. It's different from living alone over there. But even so, if I live alone, I would still make food for myself.

What are your thoughts about mask wearing?

Everyone should wear a mask, regardless if you feel sick or not. If you don't wear it for yourself then at least wear it out of respect for others, because you may be a carrier.

Can you explain what it's like in Cambodia, about people wearing masks compared to Lowell since you have experiences in both places?

The people also wear masks, and it's almost socially frowned upon if you don't wear masks. And people were here; lately, the cases have gone up. But before, there were zero cases, none over here. So, people were getting cocky. They weren't wearing masks at all. They were still going to the malls, arcades, partying, weddings, and no one was wearing a mask. Even now we have like nine cases. No one is still wearing any masks. They just don't think of it as a big deal as it really is.

Do you, yourself, wear masks when you go out in Cambodia?

Yeah, I still wear masks. Even when I'm working out or running or doing all that stuff, I still wear a mask. I don't care if they don't. I'm still going to wear it.

Are there any guidelines in Cambodia?

There are guidelines here. There are signs all over the place saying, "If you don't wear a mask, you cannot enter." Some stores really enforce that, and some stores don't. And there's also, like in Market Basket, you have to stand six feet apart. They have stickers placed on the floor, at the checkout lines. We have those too at the malls. Some people follow it. Some people don't. Most people don't because they just don't care anymore.

Have you received a Covid test and if you did, how did that go?

I received the Covid test twice: once when I landed, and then another time after fourteen days of my quarantine. It's just a simple test—they put a Q-tip up my nose and then another one down my throat. And then within one or two days you can call a number that tells you the results and then they'll just let you know.

How have things been for you in terms of being clean? Pre-pandemic and now, is there anything different you've done?

So, there hasn't been anything much different from before just because I'm me. I was brought up to be really like, almost a clean freak. I would always leave hand sanitizer in my car as default already. And whenever I go out and come back home, I just wash my hands, wash everything before I touch anything else. That habit is already embedded in me. And this virus is just making me more aware that oh, maybe I am too clean. Like this isn't normal. Um, but aside from that nothing really changed since it already is part of my day-to-day habits.

What do you think the city of Lowell and/or the federal government can or should do to keep residents safe and healthy during the pandemic?

It's a really simple thing to stay safe and healthy. Just respect the guidelines that the authorities have given out. Because every-one takes it to heart that it's a free country, you can't really restrict everyone too much. You can only enforce them so much until they start rebelling. Even suggesting a mask to them, they already start to protest. So, I can only imagine how difficult it is for them to actually come up with any sure-fire way to help everyone protect themselves. So, that question I don't think I can answer.

What about Cambodia?

Cambodian culture is much different from American culture. As I have mentioned before, America really values freedom and over here, people fear. And the government uses that to their advantage. They would show on the news, "Oh hey, you could die, or this could happen if you don't do this." People start to panic; people start to fear. And within the first few days, when the virus first started, the streets were completely empty. Here, people are much more afraid to die than people in America, I guess.

So you think in Cambodia, that the government will take more mea-sures to help keep people safe?

Yeah, definitely. It's only been nine cases and already the gov-ernment is shutting down theaters and karaokes again.

Has it affected your family life?

Um, well, we've stocked up on masks and alcohol, because, like, over there [U.S.], alcohol and toilet paper is gone. Over here [Cambodia], people hoard masks and alcohol. The mask prices here skyrocket so fast.

Do you want to talk any more about your experiences with the move?

The move? It happened really fast. I would just spend all my wak-ing hours packing my stuff. And when I slept, I'd be exhausted.

During the moving day, a lot of complications happened, but because all the decisions were decided at the last minute, I had to do everything within those two days to move all my stuff and make it to my flight on time that night. So, it was just a really hectic week, I'd say.

Was there any fear about traveling?

That was one of my fears about going, but if it's something that's already been decided, there's no point in being afraid.

Did you take any more precautions or safety measures when you flew?

Well, I had a friend flying with me and he had like a whole supply of alcohol and lotion. So, we helped each other out, and we just relied on masks and alcohol. What more can we do? Just staying away from other people and all that.

Were there a lot of people on your flight?

No. The airline did a pretty good job keeping people far away. Each person had their own row. It's almost like you're flying first class. So, you get all those three chairs to yourself. But there were some people on the flight that took their masks off while they were sleeping. It was a sixteen-hour flight. I sort of don't blame them because that is sort of suffocating to sleep with a mask on; even I was suffocated. But I still kept mine on.

You also said that you were in quarantine. Can you explain what that was like?

So, the process here, when you get the first test, everyone on the plane gets tested and we all get put into a hotel. If the test results come back and no one on that flight has anything, then we are released to go back home. But we have the responsibility to stay inside our home for fourteen days. And it's also a responsibility of us and the house members to get a retest after fourteen days.

So, everyone in your house had to get a test too?

It's not required. But everyone, I guess, was confident that they didn't need a test, or they were scared to get a test. So, they didn't get one. But I got one. And luckily for them, and me, I came out negative.

When are you planning to come back to Lowell? Are you waiting for the virus to be over?

Originally, my return flight was set for January 6, 2021. It's now been pushed further because the virus doesn't seem to be going anywhere. And my family will only allow me to go back if everything settles down over there.

How do you feel about that?

Annoyed. Of course, I want to go back. And I've been there so I feel like it's not that big. It is a big deal, but it's not major to the point where I'm like escaping war.

Do you feel safer in Cambodia?

They (the family) feel safer that I'm here. But I feel no safer here than I am over there.

Can you explain why?

Over there, I live by myself so there's less chance of me catching anything from anyone else. And I know how to take care of myself over there. It's not like I go out every single day.

***

Update

I've returned to the States since December 2021 and have read-justed back to campus life. It has been difficult to try to catch up to all my friends since I've been gone for nearly two years. The most dramatic change since coming back was readjusting back into my independent lifestyle here in the States, as opposed to my life back home where I mainly relied on my family. As of now, I am focused on my final semester and will be graduating with a bachelor's degree in management. I've been accepted into UMass Lowell's master's program in marketing and will pursue that degree as well—Sreivuthy Hak

Dear Charlotte,
You were one of
my favorite parts
of BLSE this
Summer. I loved
being in both
classes with you.
Thank you so
much for showing
up tonight in
support and for
listening to our
stories.

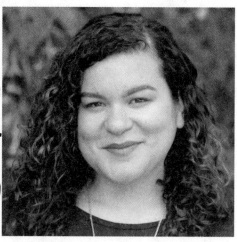

Dr. Marianela Rivera

"My community, my hometown means the world to me, it means everything to me. So if I can shine a light on a problem and try to use the gifts of education that were given to me, use my privilege as an educated Latina to help find the root causes to solve the issues to address these systemic issues through effective policy, that's what I need to do to help my people."

Dr. Marianela Rivera is a thirty-five-year-old woman who describes her ethnicity as Puerto Rican. She tells the story of her run for state representative in 2020 and her activism for educational reform, community empowerment, and racial equity. She holds a doctorate in physical therapy from Northeastern University and is currently the Public Education Organizer for Massachusetts Jobs for Justice.

Marianela was interviewed by Phillips Academy students Saffron A. and Lily R. on May 3, 2021.

What is your occupation?

Well, I am a physical therapist, but I would also describe myself as a radical activist and organizer, that's a part of what I do.

What influenced your decision to run for state representative? Could you tell us a little about your campaign, and which issues you find most important?

My run for state rep was really motivated by the fear and anxiety I had about how Covid-19 would impact education. It was rooted in the fear of disaster capitalism and the "shock doctrine" and understanding the impact that the disaster of Hurricane Katrina had on New Orleans public schools. So my fear was like, Oh my gosh, it's always in the midst of a disaster that we have all these crazy policies that are passed because people aren't paying attention, people are so focused on surviving in the middle of a pandemic that there's no opportunity to really keep track of what our representatives are doing with the State House. I had also just personally experienced how corrupt our government was while seated on the education committee, just by the interactions I had with the secretary and the commissioner, seeing how disempowered we were as a community. I felt like I needed to run to try to disrupt the corrupt political status quo. And also, when I looked back at my experiences while I was on the school committee, I realized that the systemic issues were coming from state policy, and that if I really wanted to change things for Lawrence and other communities like Lawrence I needed to be a part of the legislature and be a part of amending and repealing some of these laws.

The reason we're under receivership is because a state law was passed allowing the Board of Education to strip the Lawrence School Committee of their governing power and disempower our local teacher's union. And so, I felt like if I was gonna do anything about this issue, I had to tackle it at the root cause. Again, that really is coming from my brain as a physical therapist—when I'm treating the patient and they're complaining about back pain, I have to find what the root cause of that pain could be, and it could be a multitude of things, and so for me, it was important to go to the root cause of the problem and attack it as a source. And so I felt that if I became a state rep that I would have the opportunity to sponsor a bill to change the law that disenfranchised us.

So, it was a combination of concern over what could happen because of disaster capitalism, but then also, I had walked away from my second term on the school committee fully dedicated to being the table coordinator for the Greater Lawrence Education Justice Alliance and continuing my activism and community organizing work that way. But this was an opportunity for me to continue to spread awareness as to what was happening in our educational system, and then also the transparency issue at the State House, which not a lot of people were talking about until the 2020 races. That's why I ran for state rep. I was just honestly, reflecting one day—and it was a last-minute run. Most people who run for state rep announce their run a year before, and they do all this fancy stuff, and for me, it was more like, Well, we're in the middle of a pandemic, they just decreased the signature requirement for state rep, who's running right now? What's gonna happen? And so it was all these questions and concerns that I had that ultimately led me to pull papers two weeks before signatures were due and get on the ballot.

And I did, and I'm really proud of the fact that I did that. It was something new, something I had never experienced before and I learned a lot through it, and I met a lot of really cool people. I think if I could go back in time, I would just do it all over again the way I did it, even though I lost, because I think it's important for a healthy democracy that there are more primaries. In Massachusetts, we don't really see that a lot. We don't see a lot of people getting primaried, and I honestly think that's really important. Pass the baton, you know what I mean?

You clearly are passionate about Lawrence and its future. What are you working on right now, other than being a physical therapist?

Right now, I am the Public Education Organizer for Massachu-setts Jobs for Justice. I am really excited about this opportunity. I just started working for the organization two months ago. I had to take a break from public education. I was working for Peabody Public Schools, but honestly in the midst of a pandemic with all of the bureaucracy, everything that was going on in education and just feeling unsafe within the schools, and just like the fear I had in coming home and getting my mom, who's high-risk, sick with Covid, I was just so scared. So I was looking for an opportu-nity where I could work from home and be able to support my son who's learning remotely from home, and just keep everybody safe, and this opportunity came up to work for Jobs for Justice. And one of the executive directors who reached out to me about this opportunity, she was well aware of my work in Lawrence doing education advocacy and activism work, and she felt that I would be perfect for the position. She highly encouraged me to apply and at first, I was like, no, I'm not gonna do that, I'm a physical therapist, I think I want to do my physical therapy thing. But when I looked into the job description and what I'd be working on state-wide, it just really aligned with my passion for justice, and I felt that maybe doing something different in the midst of the pandemic might be re-energizing and refreshing.

I was really burning out working in special education. At the start of the school year, I was completely behind because of the school closure due to the lockdown, and so I just felt like I was drowning. I could never catch up with my work and my students were the ones who were suffering, because instead of hiring another therapist to help catch up on the evaluation and the services that were missed, they just expected us to do it ourselves. And with one physical therapist for the entire district, which didn't make sense. But now, as an organizer for Jobs for Justice, I get to work on building coalitions throughout the state to address education justice issues in different communities. My job is to conduct a landscape assessment and understand what the current coalitions look like in terms of justice and helping them expand while also creating three new tables that are like Greater Lawrence Education Justice Alliance throughout the state. I've met parent-activists and leaders across the state, and I've met some really awesome youth from Belchertown that started a student union in the middle of the pandemic as a result of the Black Lives Matter movement and seeing everything unfold. They felt that they needed to do their own work within their school to help students of color. And so they started this really cool union, and we've developed a relationship, and I'm trying to expand that union.

You described yourself as a radical. What does that mean to you?

So I kind of took that term—the term of radical—which was really weaponized and used against me when I was doing my advocacy work on the school committee, and I transformed it into something positive. I gotta thank Dr. Angela Davis for it, because I remember seeing a quote in which she says radical simply means grasping things at the root, and I was like, Yeah, that's exactly what I'm doing. I'm trying to find what are the root causes of these problems and I'm trying to address it for my community. My community, my hometown means the world to me, it means everything to me, and so if I can shine a light on a problem and try to use the gifts of education that were given to me, use my privilege as an educated Latina help find the root causes to solve the issues and address these systemic issues through effective policy, that's what I need to do to help my people. Now, before I used to think it was this negative term being used against me, and now I'm just like, no, I'm proud of it, and I say that I'm a radical activist because I am always going to try to find the root cause of the problem and help my people in the best way that I can. If that upsets people in power, so be it. If people in power or try to discredit me, defame me, do whatever they feel is necessary to stop my activist work, that's fine, but I'm gonna continue to be a radical. I definitely am proud of the fact that I use my voice and I use my intelligence to help my community out, and I will use that term from here on out in a positive light.

***

Update

I've been keeping myself very busy during the pandemic. Keeping busy has been a coping mechanism to distract me from all the anxiety around the pandemic and the global chaos. After the interview, I was accepted into the Perrone Sizer Institute for Creative Leadership and in the EforAll Lowell Winter 2022 Business Accelerator program. I started a physical therapy and wellness coaching business along with an education consultancy business with Kassandra Infante. We want to use our experience in education and politics to help schools and non-profits with Diversity, Equity, Inclusion and Justice (DEIJ) efforts and civic education. Our hope is to start a foundation for education justice and one day open up a school in Lawrence—Dr. Marianela Rivera

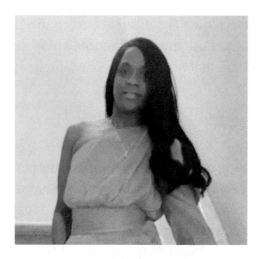

Cristie Galíndez

"I gave my one hundred percent and more, and tried every day to improve how to teach each student through this pandemic"

Cristie Galíndez is a forty-one-year-old Hispanic woman from Puerto Rico. She is a crisis paraprofessional and has been a teacher's assistant for fourteen years. For the last five years, she has worked in the field of Spanish enrichment and computers for school children. She oversees teaching children in Spanish at John Breen School in Lawrence, Mass.

Note – The original interview was conducted in Spanish. This is an English translation.

Cristie was interviewed by Phillips Academy students Gloria C., Carly P., and Diego E. (her son) on May 2, 2021.

How did Covid-19 affect the students?

I feel that Covid-19 affected the students a lot, especially the grade I teach. We had several weeks without classes, so a lot of education was lost. There are a lot of parents I know who worked with the students in their house. Many did not, and it is understood it was something that nobody expected, nobody knew about this crisis that we had. So whatever was going on in different homes we understood. And since it was in the middle of the pandemic we had to do the classes through Zoom, which was, in my opinion, something horrible. When teaching a five or six year old how to use a pencil, how to sound out words . . . it helps to be present so that children can learn. I feel that this Covid-19 greatly delayed education, especially for parents who did not know technology. Many parents do not know technology, some did not, some yes. The materials that we need—some had them in the house while others did not. There were many, many problems that we were not prepared for.

What do you think about using Zoom?

Personally, I'm learning every day because I'm still having class through Zoom—we have part in person and part still on Zoom, and every day I'm learning something new. I didn't know any-thing about this; I don't know how to work with it, etc., but I had to learn quite a few things about Zoom, since it was all on there. I had to send them documents, to teach the children, to give them things. It was boring, because I know that kids love electronics in front of their face and also playing and things like that, but Zoom is different. Kids are sitting for two hours, two and a half hours, whatever the time is that we have now. That's why there's also a teacher in front of the Zoom. Sometimes without anything more than looking, looking, looking it can become very difficult, but we were preparing ourselves with different tools to use with Zoom so that we could make the class a little more fun, so that they could participate more and it would seem more or less as in person, but through the computer.

You talked about doing things so that your students draw their atten-tion to you. How did Zoom affect the students' attention?

It affected them a lot. We tried to teach for at least ten to twenty minutes, give a break or a recess time or put on music or stretches or playing with them, converse with them. They love it, and it makes the class a little more fun, because a four-year-old child says, "Why do I have to sit for so long?" It is very difficult, so we try to have enough recess so that they felt a little more comfortable and it wasn't so boring or so intense for them to be sitting in a chair for so many hours looking at the computer through Zoom.

Do you think that the plan of John Breen School and Covid-19 worked well or do you think it could have been something different?

I feel that the John Breen School worked very well. I feel that I did a good job because it was something that everyone was learning. It was not something that I had any experience with, nobody has the experience about how to teach a child in the middle of this pandemic. So day by day we were improving, I mean, I don't know, in my opinion we were improving, we were trying, we tried to do the best that each one of us could, and we kept learning because we still haven't finished. If we still manage to use Zoom and we try to do this as calmly as possible, the more fun, the easier it is for them to feel comfortable. Because I know that the pandemic affected many places and we don't know exactly how it felt in each family. So we were pretty flexible with everything with the whole family and tried to understand each individual child.

Since Covid went on for a long time, when was the most difficult time for you?

Many teachers thought that it was going to be for a short time and when we saw that it was more days, and the months went by, it made it a little more difficult. We did many activities with the children, but the time was in front of a computer. We did not do any activity that we normally did during the year. I think that was a bit difficult and sad since every year I always look for what we are going to do next with these students, what are the activities that we are going to plan for another year. Seeing these activities that we planned a year before that we did not do, we say wow. We planned all this for nothing. And I feel that many of the teachers think the same as I did. We said that we plan so many activities, so many things for a student and then it vanishes because we can't do anything. So, I feel that those things were difficult since we don't know how long this will be, so we still have to get used to Covid-19 and the pandemic to teach students in this way. So, I'm planning one day at a time. I'm no longer thinking ahead with this pandemic, because you don't know what's going to happen yet.

How can you connect to your students in the classroom or remote learning?

In my opinion, to have that connection with each individual student, I like to observe each student, to know what they like, to know what they don't like. I observe their physical form, what makes them angry; remotely, you can't see any of that. In the middle of a screen sometimes you can only see from their little eyes and upward, and they are sitting and you can't see them over on the side. So you have to be flexible with it, you can give yourself the time. I'm saying "Juan, stand in front of the camera," because they don't like it very much, so we try to be flexible. And then to have that connection with the student, it is difficult. I don't know. What we are doing on Zoom, is not like having a separate room to take the kids aside to get to know them and talk to each other about any topic. I feel that this year I did not have that connection with the students in individual groups since through Zoom it is very difficult, I think at any age, but at four and five years old it is very difficult. I also think because there are only two grades in the school, they had not had that connection before because they didn't have a lot of time with each child.

What do you think you learned during this pandemic?

I think that Covid has taught me to have a lot of patience. Since it is super difficult to teach a child over the computer, this has been horrible in my opinion, so I feel that Covid has taught me to be patient, to take every day one at a time. Trying to be flexible with the different families, since we didn't know what each other was going through, so I tried to be flexible with myself as well. Not to feel frustrated since I or some child couldn't join the class, the internet wasn't working, the internet shut off. I said, fine, I am doing the best I can, giving one hundred percent of myself and trying to continue, to not beat myself up, and do my best.

Do you have something to say to other teachers about teaching during the pandemic?

They should not be hard on themselves. I know that I have many colleagues who felt frustrated because they feel that this year, we did not teach the students enough, but I feel that what was happening with the pandemic no one was expecting, and we have to be patient and say to ourselves that we did the best we could, since it was something new and nobody expected it. That it isn't easy, but nobody knew of this, so I try to be fair with myself and say, Well I'm going to do the best I can. I know it's not going to be easy, but we have to keep going, and if we like to be teachers, we have to keep going. We cannot beat ourselves up and say— get frustrated. Personally, I got quite frustrated one time, but I learned that it was something new, it was something that I did not expect and many did not expect. And speaking for myself, I gave my one hundred percent and more, and tried every day to improve how to teach each student through this pandemic.

What do you think about the education system in Lawrence today?

I know that this was something new that was not there before, that it was unexpected, but I feel that they could have prepared us a little better. Since many, many, many, many teachers were very frustrated, because they didn't know how to manage Zoom, they didn't know how to share pages or the assignments for the students. Many things I think I know, but I think that they should have prepared it a little better, a little better. A number of us knew what we were doing, some of us learned by looking up tutorials on YouTube, it was not something that they taught us, but that you had to learn by yourself. And I feel that in that sense, the Lawrence schools or the education department failed us a little bit there. I feel that they didn't have to teach us more, but that they should have prepared us more for that.

We are not perfect in Lawrence schools, but we are working so hard to have a better future for the children. I know that they are working hard. Every day I see that they are fixing bad schools and bringing more and more educational programs for the students, so I feel that they are working hard to move Lawrence and Lawrence Public Schools forward and for children to have a better future.

***

Update

I continue to work in the same school, giving my best for the future of my students. In my opinion, the pandemic challenged the best of me as a teacher; working within the pandemic, I did not see it as more work, but as an opportunity to learn and teach in a different way. While I was teaching, I realized my ability and the love I have for my work—Cristie Galíndez

2.

Providing Healthcare: Rehabilitation Centers and Nursing Homes

Tom Coppinger
Director of the Point After Club in Lawrence, a rehabilitation center for people with mental illnesses

Xavier Robbins
Dancer, graphic designer, and care worker at a rehabilitation center in Lowell

Miranda Melo
UMass Lowell alumna, Registered Nurse in Lowell

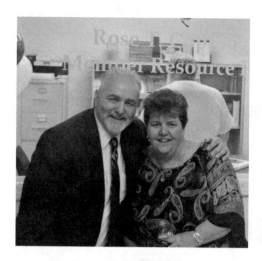

Tom Coppinger

"Every day is a new day and what really gives me hope is that within this community here that we work with, there's the Point After Club community. I have the most tremendous staff and members that a person could ever want, people really care and love each other."

Tom Coppinger is the director of the Point After Club in Lawrence, a rehabilitation center started in 1982. The club provides rehabilitation services to people with mental illnesses. Tom has met the challenges of the pandemic with hard work and determination, continuing to provide the club's services to people in need. He is sixty-three years old and describes himself as Irish-American.

Tom was interviewed by Phillips Academy students Amelia V. and Henry C. on May 8, 2020.

My full name is Thomas Gabriel Coppinger Sr. I have a Junior. I was born December 30, 1956, at the Holy Family Hospital, known as the Bon Secour back then, in Methuen. My hometown growing up was Salem, New Hampshire. I'm currently residing, for the last twenty years, in Westford, Mass. In fact, we have a purchase and sale on our house right now, which is pretty exciting—my wife's family home. And I am the director of the Point After Club, which is a rehabilitation program here in Lawrence. We're gonna talk about that a lot. I've been with the club, as of June 15th, for forty years.

What is the mission of the Point After Club?

My mother Rose T. Coppinger founded the Club in 1980 so discharged patients from Danvers State Hospital would have a place to belong and be accepted and appreciated for who they are. And in the process, work towards developing opportunities to better their lives. I went to Luckenbach, Texas in 1982. There's a song out there "everybody is somebody in Luckenbach," and I came back in 1982 and we kind of adopted that at the Point After Club. Everybody is somebody at the Point After Club. I think that's something we are extremely proud of and something that my mother always drove in—everyone's life is important and everyone's got a story in life. Her mother even told her prior to that, "Give people an opportunity to be . . . take them for who you see them as, with fresh eyes." And I think that is something that we have lived with at the Club, as a part of our philosophy since our beginning. And you know, sometimes it's amazing that some of these folks are walking through the door with the stories that they come in with. The resiliency is incredible, but instead of judging them, you know, support them. See what we can do to help them move forward in their lives, just like what everyone else needs. You know, a decent place to live, a job—meaningful work, meaningful opportunity, meaningful relationships, you know—friendships.

When you asked about our mission, we're a part of what is now an international rehabilitation model, the clubhouse model of rehabilitation where our standards came out in 1989 and we offer our members four guaranteed rights: a place to come, meaningful work, meaningful relationships, and a place to return. So it's a community, it's an intentional community to give a place that they can come but isn't a silo, not a place that we just come in here and create a mini institution ourselves, you know, come out of the hospitals, but a place that is part of the community. And I've never been more proud of us as I am now during this pandemic because of the community connections that we have developed over the years and because our clubhouse community has a larger community that plays a huge role in our success as members move forward in their recovery.

How has the pandemic forced you to change your operations?

My mother would be the first one to say, "I do not do this myself, I have an incredible staff." I've gathered so many different people over the years, including my wife because she worked for us before. Of course, I didn't go out with her when she was working—she ended up coming and working for the club.

In 2020, on March 17th we were having our corned beef and cabbage dinner. We normally have about seventy people for our corned beef and cabbage dinner. We have a jug band, we play all the Irish songs, you know—it's one of our big celebrations. That Saturday it was our friends and family event which is great. We have three major friends and family events to bring family members into the clubhouse and they can show their pride for their club. We'll break bread and we'll sing songs, and we'll have fun.

March 17th was the day we were told that March 18th we were going to be shutting down for any on-site operations. Also, the governor had said there could not be any groups of twenty-five or larger. We told people we weren't gonna do the corned beef and cabbage. However, we still had like forty-something people. I was in a conference call about emergency, you know, and how this is all gonna play out and it was very, very difficult because from one day we're running our operations, everybody's coming in—so we have a working routine, we have a morning meeting, you know, so what's happening today, quote of the day, standard of the week, who's doing what, let's appreciate so-and-so for their jobs, shout outs, and so forth. Then we have unit meetings, who's gonna do what. We have it on whiteboards. Members say "I'm gonna do this," and members volunteer everyday in the unit meetings about what they're gonna be doing. So there's this routine. We have lunch between 12 p.m. and 1 p.m., then back to work. We're doing reach-out now, let's go check in on other jobs in the community and other things. So all of a sudden the next day, we're closed! We have no work order day, and our members can't come. It was, Oh my god, what are we gonna do?

We did see it coming, somewhat. We were a little bit proactive. I spoke with what's called the ACCS, the Adult Clinical Community Services, they're our partners and colleagues with our agency Vinfen Corp. They do the community mental health. I spoke with Kristi who used to be my boss with the clubhouses. She is the Regional Manager for Vinfen and works with them while looking to support people in case of this type of a closure. One of the things we knew that we could do, we have a beautiful kitchen, we built out a beautiful kitchen. We're in the Everett Mills now and I just have to mention Marianne Paley Nadel, the owner of the building, and Tom Brown, they were incredible. And we have this tremendous space that we designed, which we're so proud of. I said, "We have the kitchen," this was a week before then, "when this closes down we will have the capacity to make meals. That's one thing we can do." We know people are reliant on that meal. Some folks are living in rooming houses, you know, they have nowhere they can find cooking. We live in a great community as far as supporting people, but Bread and Roses, one of the soup kitchens, closed down. And, you know, some folks really have a hard time going out—based on the nature of their symptoms too, which can make it very difficult for them. A lot of folks relied on that meal that we had at the club. We were ready to go on Wednesday. We knew that Wednesday the 18th that this was something we could do.

However, you know, getting this message out to everybody . . . and then we're wired to engage our members as part of our job, you know, I was talking to someone "Why don't you come to the club!?" But I can't say that anymore. You can't because we're closed for on-site operation, and we're trying to think of ways we can still be a clubhouse, a virtual clubhouse, you know, this is part of this. We've been introduced to Zoom, we've been doing Zoom meetings and it's awesome. This is something we've adapted to. We will continue to adapt to as best we can, but it was . . . probably the most challenging—you know, I've never been more proud of this club. I mean my staff have been off the charts. I mean we're out there delivering meals—they basically, you know, will do anything.

As time progressed, we were asked to reduce the number of staff that could be on-site to reduce the risk that we're contaminating each other with this terrible virus. But my staff have been so incredibly energetic and positive and doing the job, making the meals, delivering the meals, making the phone calls. So we started massive reach-out everyday. We're calling our members everyday. Check-ins, what's going on, you know. We're helping people with their stimulus checks.

We have many members working. You know, there's thirty-six clubhouses in Massachusetts—last year we were the number one in clubs in competitive employment. We had thirty-four percent of our members in employment. For six months out of the year we've been in the top five all months, which we're very proud of. Here in the city of Lawrence we have one of the higher unemployment rates in the state, but because we work here, it's part of our culture, we see the importance of it. Again that's my staff, and the members too, working to support each other.

And now it's the challenge of people losing their jobs. We still have a lot of members that are working, and we just went over the list yesterday of the members that are still working whether it's at Stop & Shop, Market Basket, Family Dollar. We've got a member that works at the Independent Living Center, and we had a member that just went back to a company to make masks. This company has just diverted to making masks. And through this process, we know that maintaining positive relationships and supporting each other has been the core, the most import-ant thing for us. And it's more than the meal. When you deliver a meal, these members are coming out, you can see, like the relationship is there, the gratitude. They're helping us. And then as we go through this, we got members that want to make meals, they want to help people with rides. They want to help out too, which is very, very difficult because we also know the stay-at-home order is there for a reason. And we don't want anybody getting sick. We've got to be vigilant ourselves with masks and with gloves, you know, we've been fortunate.

My sister-in-law Sue and a friend of hers, Patty, made a bunch of masks for us right off the bat. Debbie's Treasure Chest here in the building hooked us up with National Fiber Tech-nology in Everett Mills and they make these masks, they're really cool. They make a mask and donate a mask. Yesterday the Salvation Army gave us broccoli, lettuce, and celery, you know, organic. We're getting stuff out of Boston, free food. Merrimack Valley Food Bank has been an incredible support. We just got a really long list of community partners that we work with. I hate to miss out names when I start talking about how many people—the MSPCA is giving us dog food and cat food for our members' cats and dogs. It's just incredible. Chicken Connec-tion from Haverhill donated a meal. They made sixty meals for us last Wednesday, we didn't have to cook that day. We just picked them up and delivered the meals. The Adult Community Clinical Services (ACCS) folks are delivering about twenty-five meals a day and we're delivering about thirty-five, so we're partnering with them so the meals are big.

But we still got to figure out how are we gonna do this. We've been doing virtual meetings, and we find that that's a challenge too because a lot of members do not have smartphones. Before this we were working with Beth Israel and Harvard with smartphone training, and we actually got some members smartphones. So this was kind of ironic the way this happened. Some of our members were being trained for this. I know I've done virtual meetings before but now I'm hosting some of these meetings, which is a nightmare. The pandemic itself, as I said, has taken us to another level.

May 1st we were supposed to have our annual mental health awareness event. We use the Mental Health America format. We have an art gallery open for the month of May, it's Mental Health Awareness Month, and we had to cancel that. But what we're doing now is we're gonna do it. Like I contacted the mayor's office, I spoke with his chief of staff Kate, you know, and I said, "We want the mayor to proclaim it Mental Health Awareness Month." I gave her the template and we want to have him do that. He's done it the last six years, we've been doing this for six years. We have members—we have the format . . . we've been giving the members the format and this is about, you know, toxic influences and stuff, owning your feelings, some really good stuff, but it's about tools to thrive. Things that can help you thrive in your life, so we're giving that stuff out. UMass Nutrition Extension program has given us a weekly newsletter with Covid related stuff . . . that is very positive.

We're gonna do a virtual mental health awareness event having the mayor claim it—mental health awareness, but it's engaging our members, you know they say they're so bored they want to get back to the club. We want them, we need them back at the club in order to do what we are doing, but this is really bringing the community together. And you can really feel it, they're excited and it's pretty obvious that this isn't going to be over tomorrow, you know that we're in this for the long run. We are adopting more virtual meetings. We had a virtual employment one and we're going to at least do a virtual meeting daily focusing on health and wellness, all the stuff we do, the communications in housing and stuff. We're still involved in virtual meetings with the State Mental Health Planning Council on housing and the Massachusetts Clubhouse Coalition. For the Clubhouse Coalition, we are the chairs of the advocacy committee. We put out a statement about all the things the clubhouse is doing at this time as well as our legislators, we want them to know that we're funded through Massachusetts taxpayers' dollars, they're getting their dollars' worth. We are not curling up, you know, we are here, we have a commitment to our membership and making sure they are ok. I think that's where we are at and understand it is not easy but we're doing it.

Is there anything you are doing now in the Point After Club that you had to do because of the pandemic, that you might continue once things return to normal?

Well, I think it was Albert Einstein who said, "In the midst of difficulties lie opportunities." I think what we are seeing clearly is that wow, when you are in the middle of something, when you are able to work, when we're at the club it's just like we're off the charts, we're on and every day has its own story. And so you kind of have these plans, we do have these planning days to make the objective that we're a very accomplished clubhouse. We've gotten a three-year unconditional accreditation since 1998. I mean that's remarkable. A lot of clubs have challenges with that, but we're an incredible community. However, it's hard to accomplish certain things. We've been talking about a Facebook page for a long time and we now have a tremendous Facebook page that just started after March 18th, Point After Clubhouse, check it out, it's pretty cool. There's a lot of resources on that, but we see it as an opportunity moving forward. I guess the urgency around people learning about technology, our members and staff, you know this virtual stuff, and how this is an opportunity. We even talked about one of the groups we really want to reach out to—you know, our major goal is to get young adults more involved in the clubhouse. We have a young adult program across the hall from us and they are more in tune to this type of stuff, but gathering groups of people virtually is a lot easier, you know, if you have the savvy and knowledge on how to do it.

But these virtual meetings with other clubhouses, you know with our coalition, this is huge. We talked about doing it but it's one of those things you never really did, you know you'd have phone calls so you hear the voice, this changes when we talk to somebody. It really does change the whole spirit of the meeting, and we see this as another tremendous opportunity. Even WhatsApp, our members are learning all kinds of things too so that we can communicate with them. And we've been working on the new database, making sure we get everybody's email address, and if they don't have one we are going to try to help them get one. Teaching people that type of stuff, I think would benefit us moving forward significantly.

What gives you hope in terms of the pandemic, for mental health, and in general?

What gives me hope is that every day is a new day and what really gives me hope is within this community, the Point After Club community, I have the most tremendous staff and members that a person could ever want, you know people really care and love each other. It means so much that we have been through the highs and the lows together, and everybody really roots for each other and that's really important. But also, this wonderful city of Lawrence, I think there was no community prepared for this more than the city of Lawrence. The non-profits that we work with and other folks were ready to go, ready to take this on and support each other. I don't live in the city of Lawrence, but

I certainly love it and have spent a lot of my time in the city of Lawrence over the last forty years, and I have a lot of hope for the future. I have a lot of hope when I see people—their generosity. Sometimes it's people that don't have anything that want to give, and they will and it's very good. I'm just very hopeful.

***

Update

The Point After Club Community has overcome many adversities over the years, and the pandemic has brought out the best in all of us. It has been almost two years since my interview, and I can honestly say I couldn't be any prouder of the members and staff of the Club. Our clubhouse community faced our biggest challenge ever, and with the support of our community partners and our agency Vinfen we continue to work together to develop meaningful opportunities for our membership. During the pandemic we delivered over 30,000 meals to members of the club, and we know it was a lot more than the meal we were delivering. We ran a vaccine clinic on February 25, 2021, and a second one on March 25, 2021. We learned about Zoom, Microsoft Teams, Webex, FaceTime, WhatsApp, and went from a virtual clubhouse to a hybrid. These are tools that have proven to be invaluable. Our clubhouse's biggest strength has always been our ability to maintain positive relationships and support each other in the best and worst times. This resilient attitude has never been more evident than in these past two years dealing with everything this pandemic has thrown at us. I believe that we are almost done with the worst of this pandemic and feel confident that better times are ahead for us all—Tom Coppinger

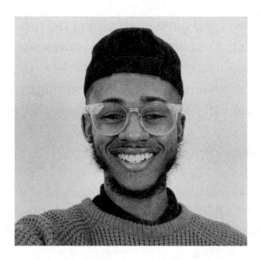

Xavier Robbins

"I've learned so much during this season of Covid. I've learned so much about fear. I've learned so much about not letting fear consume me and kind of looking at the positivity in everything and putting my trust in God's word and what God says in his word."

Xavier Robbins is a twenty-three-year-old graphic designer and break dancer who describes his ethnicity as Trinidadian/Native American. He has lived with his family in Lowell for the past nine years. During the pandemic, he created a new business customizing shoes and also was an essential care worker at a rehabilitation center for the elderly. Xavier discusses challenges he and his family members faced both at work and at home, and how his faith in God helped him cope.

Xavier was interviewed by Rebecca Phillips on November 12, 2020.

What is your story, how has this pandemic impacted you?

Besides being a graphic designer, I am also a break-dancer. I have been dancing with Phunk Phenomenon. We were on a roll with getting shows, doing gigs, getting paid for a lot of the performances. We were actually supposed to fly out to Arizona for one of the world's biggest hip-hop competitions ever. And this was going to be my first time doing that. We were actually going to be performing there, besides competing. But all of that excitement, hard work, time, and dedication practicing for this global event got stopped because of Covid. When Covid came, the dance studio completely shut down. We were struggling with getting all of our students and team members on video calls for practices, alongside with Covid impacting us in the dance community. It impacted our studio significantly, because we lost a lot of our prime members who have been on the team for two to three years. A lot of people dropped out of the dance company because they had to focus on their health issues and making sure they're safe first. It kind of discouraged me that I trained for a whole year with them and it kind of just went down the drain. We actually don't know when we will be able to go back out there or even get invited to go back out there to perform. So, that is one thing that really impacted me during Covid, because I love to dance. Covid also impacted just being free, just having the free will.

Oh quarantine, quarantine life.

I definitely understand the safety regulations that the state put in place for us to wear masks and to cover our face so that way saliva won't get on people and put people at risk and danger. It's just something you have to get used to. And I'm still, even now, getting used to putting a mask on my face, sometimes I tend to forget to put it on. They have to tell me to put it on. Rather than that, Covid just really messed up the dance for me and practices. I would go to break dance practices in Lowell, locally.

When did you start that?

I started going to this place to practice called United Teen Equality Center (UTEC) when I first moved to Lowell about nine years ago. So, I've been going there for nine years consecutively, like every day. After middle school, after high school, after college. Not going there anymore for such a long period of time was odd and strange. That kind of messed up the flow. I had to adjust and move stuff around in my house. I moved my bed in my room, so I can have a little bit more space to do some type of dance. It worked out pretty well.

How has your routine changed?

In the beginning of Covid at least, my schedule became a lot clearer, because I wasn't going to dance rehearsals. I didn't have to attend my breakdance practices on the weekdays with my crew. So it was literally just work, go home and pretty much do freelance graphic design on the side and I've always pretty much been doing that. Although, Covid gave me a lot more free time to actually focus on graphic design. Because I wasn't going to dance practices, it gave me more time to focus on my art. It actually helped me get into customizing shoes and I never customized shoes before, until 2020.

Wow! So, I guess this opened up a door for your creative side. How's that been going?

It's been going really well. Actually, it started off really cool, I never thought about customizing shoes, ever. A friend of mine, he's like my brother, his name's Will. We go to a church called Grace Nation. It's an amazing place, I love it so much. And my brother Will was like, "Hey man, you know, our Pastor's birthday is coming up and we know he likes shoes a lot. It'll be cool if we did a custom shoe for him." Just the thought of it . . . I was like, Yeah, we gotta do this! And when he asked me to customize the shoes, I was excited, but I was honest and let him know that I never customized shoes before. I'm a pretty good artist but never put my art on a shoe. So, long story short, he gave me a pair of his shoes. I did a custom on them and it came out horrible. He was like, "Yo man, we are going to need you to figure this out, because his birthday is coming up and you're the only guy that can really do it." So, I ended up going out and buying the shoes and looked up tutorials on how to customize shoes and I followed the instructions and kind of crossed my fingers with everything and the shoe came out great! I gave those to him and his wife, so they had matching pairs of custom shoes and from there he actually gave me a business idea. That I should actually start customizing shoes as a business.

Wow, okay so this is very different . . . so, I understand the negative aspect of it, you know, wearing masks, having to quarantine, the disruption of your plans and schedule with dancing at UTEC and Phunk Phenomenon and different things you did outside in your life. But you seem to keep pushing forward and diving into new things and passions and discovery and creativity.

Wow, that's actually true. When you say that, I actually kind of think about it. You said something really powerful, you said that I . . . yeah, it's true. It kind of was the opposite for me. I experienced what everyone else experienced . . . the shut down, the quarantine, but it also pushed me to go beyond my creative limits.

And beyond your situation.

Most definitely, because this all happened in probably like three months, four months ago. And I made more money in one month . . . in a month's time, than I ever made at my job. From just customizing shoes, creating logos and flyers for people. That was definitely something I wasn't expecting and opened my eyes to let me know this is possible. Like I wouldn't have to work a nine to five for the rest of my life. I can have another stream of income just through working with my hands. I don't have to go out and buy a big building right now. Everything I do in house, in my room, and I have all the equipment that I need for now.

So you flipped this whole pandemic upside down?

Yeah, I mean this was all God, I'm a firm believer in that. I know that God has a big role in how everything is turning out in my life. With dealing with Covid, there was a challenge I did face working at a rehabilitation center for a lot of elderly people. Before Covid started I was a waiter, a floater. When Covid hit, we had to wear masks and had to stay away from the residents and actually had to do room service, which we were never trained to do. We had to learn everything very fast, because the elderly were very needy. And we need to make sure we get to them on time. They need to eat food before they take their medicine. In my work environment, it was a very fast switch to adapt and make sure that we are attending to the residents as fast as they need us. That's with food service, being nice, and letting them know what's going on in the outside world, because they are so prone to Covid because of their age. They literally didn't know what was going on and some weren't watching the news.

I witnessed a lot of residents get Covid and some died or became really ill from Covid. I'm so used to them looking healthy for their age and then I saw some of them survive Covid and look completely different. That was something I was not used to seeing, because I'm not around a lot of elderly. It put a soft spot in my heart, not like I didn't have one, but it opened my eyes. I see these people on a daily basis, more than I see my family. I work there eight hours and sometimes twelve hours a day. Covid changed my perspective on the elderly and having to care for them at such a high demand and having to do it quick. Quicker than what we already work, because it's fast paced, especially with food service.

It definitely changed the atmosphere of your work environment.

Yeah, it made me step up and take a lot of roles and tasks and opened up my eyes to not giving up even if I was frustrated with something. I'm younger and they're much older, but I need to understand that they're living in a time where a lockdown is happening. They're so concerned. I can't be selfish, I need to think about what I feel and put myself outside the box and really make sure they are okay and healthy. It was a huge change and we were not prepared with the right equipment, too. We had masks on and we were room serving and were supposed to be wearing bodysuits. And we had an issue that the dinner's food service providers weren't fully equipped with the equipment so it was very controversial, not wanting to go there to be put at risk but also having to go up there because they need food. So we ended up having a huge meeting and the nurses having to help us in the kitchen. Even the owners of the actual facility got involved. I saw them with bodysuits and masks on. They were coming in the dining rooms, checking on residents, going up to their rooms. I mean, everybody . . . not one single person was counted out . . . was helping out to do something that they weren't used to doing. 100% everyone, even the receptionists were helping us in the kitchen with getting meals out, taking meals upstairs, letting the nurses know when to come in the kitchen, when to leave the kitchen . . . .

That must have been a stressful time for you.

It was going through it, dealing with the switch of not having that right equipment and not only that, but I was fed-up with being the only person . . . me and my brother work at the same place, but being the only person in the facility that was taking it serious and not taking it as a joke, but it's hard to say. The adjustment was stressful—even having to show up at work earlier than my usual working time. That was an adjustment; I don't really like waking up too early to go to work. But there were some days I had to be at work at 5 a.m. and I usually have to be there at

6 a.m. So that means I have to wake up at 4 a.m. to be there for 5 a.m., and to stay there sometimes till 8 p.m. I had to work from 5 a.m. to 8 p.m. That was almost normal. So it was like twelve hour shifts four days out of the week and I would work Monday through Saturday.

There wasn't really a high demand like that at all until Covid came. So I worked a lot and saw a lot of people come in and leave, because they were concerned about their health with Covid and didn't want to give it to someone elderly or want to catch it either. I saw a lot of people who liked working there who were very aware of their health and left. A lot of people I was good friends with and had a good relationship with in the company left because of Covid. It's a scary time and a lot of people were protecting themselves. So, I understand why people were leaving. That became even harder for the company. That's why a lot of people had to step in to fill in those empty gaps and spots that were left. That's another reason why we had to come in early. We had to help nurses bring stuff somewhere, people from the kitchen. Yeah, it was definitely stressful trying . . . just adjusting, period. And I feel like that's for the whole world, just adjusting is such a stressful thing.

Did they have the people there take tests?

Yes, they did, the whole place had to get tested, they had the . . . I forget what it was, the army . . . the state came in. They had hazmats, bodysuits on, we had tanks outside, literally the military jeeps with all the testing kits, hazmat suits. The news was even outside. There was a huge line in the facility, everybody was in the line, everyone had to sit down in the chair, they had people in there having to get tested all at the same time.

This was all to get a test?

Yeah, it was definitely out of the norm. Like wow, we actually have people from the army and state come in here. Like, there's jeeps outside. People coming in and out of the building with white full bodysuits, asking people a lot of questions. It was something out of a movie. And I feel like it is something like out of a movie, you see movies with lockdowns. Government comes in. You see tanks, stuff everywhere. A lot of people got tested, I got tested, it came out negative, thank God. Some people got positive, some people got negative. That's just how it goes now. It was definitely something out of the norm for me to see.

How did it affect your family?

I live with my older sister and youngest brother. My mom would come over a lot. We just moved into a condo ourselves. It definitely affected us in a way. We also had to be very careful of going out a lot and coming back home and putting each other at risk of probably catching Covid. We're really chill all three of us so we were kind of just in our own zone, not really that worried about any of us getting it. We all know where we all go. I go to church, my brother goes to church, my sister goes to work.

Okay, so you guys were staying very safe.

Yeah, we were staying very safe. But it did affect our household, because my brother was working and ended up getting Covid from the job we were working at. That definitely affected the household and my sister was worried for my brother and was nervous for herself and her health as well. Even though my brother was asymptomatic—he tested positive but didn't show any Covid symptoms. So he looked fine, felt fine, said he was fine, but the test said that he had Covid. It was a weird thing. He was not sick, but the test said that he had it. So we had to take our safety precautions. He had to stay quarantined for fourteen days in his room. I wasn't home as much, but my sister completely left the house and had to go over to her friend's house.

She didn't want to get pulled out of work, because she made the most money out of all of us, so she needed to make sure she could go to work.

Oh, so she had to leave the house you guys are at together for her health's sake, safety, to keep her job.

Yep, so she can pay the bills. Me, I just stood my six-feet distance away from my brother at all times.

But you were fine when you tested because you stayed at work.

Yeah, I was at work, got tested, I was negative so I was fine. I haven't gotten Covid at all. I got tested more than once and it came out negative even being around my brother, I was negative. So, yeah I still was going to work. He was quarantined. After his quarantine, he went to go get tested and he was negative. So, everything cleared up and my sister ended up coming back to the house more often, which was funny . . . my friends that I usually break dance with were kind of scared though. Even though I told them I was negative, they were like, "we don't know, we gotta kind of stay our distance."

But it definitely impacted the house when my brother got it. My sister ended up getting it a few months later just from going to work. It's a risk everywhere. Even being at work. Out of all things, most places are shut down, but certain jobs had to stay open because of being an essential worker.

That's what your job is? You were essential?

I'm essential yeah, so I wasn't laid off or wasn't remote. I had to go in and I had to get a printed out slip just in case the police saw me driving, I would be able to give them the slip to let them know, "Hey, I'm going to work," because I am an essential worker. So my sister was an essential worker as well and she ended up getting Covid. She couldn't go to work and her job didn't pay for sick time at all and she had to file for unemployment for Covid. Her unemployment didn't come in right away, so we were worrying about how we were going to finish paying some of the bills. That was a huge thing, so we talked to our landlord, letting her know what was going on. The policy at our place was that there wasn't any consideration for late pay because of Covid. It was kind of like, you have to have the money and that's it. So that was huge and a shocker to us and we were able to manage and pay for the bills regardless still.

It was tough dealing with my brother having Covid, out of work and not getting paid. Then, my sister being out of work, not getting paid and still having bills to pay. It was hard seeing them go through that and the frustration. I got their frustration 100% and that was a challenge emotionally for me. I felt for them and their frustration and worry about how I am going to do this. This is such a thing where you have to think fast and you have to adapt quickly and they did that, which is really good. Then, my sister ended up taking the test again, she was negative so she got better from Covid.

Oh nice! What we like to hear!

Yeah, she ended up going back to work, made money. So it was definitely an emotional, empathetic time for me with all that. I'm just glad they came out negative in the end after all that. Out of all the people who got Covid, sadly some left their loved ones. There are people who get Covid but do come out okay. I think that's huge, and I think that needs to be spread a lot more— there's not just death everywhere, that's what we're hearing. People need to start talking about people who actually came out of Covid. I think that'll give people more hope and faith that they won't die and they don't have to be that scared and that you can fight it off and it's something that's not incurable or something that you cannot get over. Because there are people who have gotten over it.

Is there anything else you wanted to share with me?

Um, not really, I mean like, what I really have left to say is that it's okay to be scared, but don't let the situation take away your faith. I've learned so much during this season of Covid. I've learned so much about fear. I've learned so much about not letting fear consume me and kind of looking at the positivity in everything and putting my trust in God's word and what God says in his word. And that he never forsakes his people. He loves them and watches over them. I hope that a lot of people continue to actually pray that this blows over sooner than we think and not just hope for the worst. I can definitely say a huge influence over my life and how I was able to stay relevantly pretty calm through Covid is definitely because of my Pastor. Pastor Gerry Mickle . . . he's an amazing man of God. He definitely helped me get through this little storm that the world is in and I know he's definitely helped a lot of other people get through the hardships and stuff like that, just by preaching truth to masses of people online. Got so many testimonies of people getting over fear, so many testimonies of people saying they've come out of Covid. He's been praying for people to be healed from Covid and people have been healed from Covid in like an instant.

Okay, alright, Thank you so much Xavier Robbins.

Thank you, I appreciate it.

***

Update

Xavier Robbins is currently working as a machine technician making optical lenses for NASA and the glass mirrors for NASA space robots and satellites. He is also still customizing shoes. If you would like to order a pair, please contact him via Instagram @10fakindcusts or email: 10fakindcustomz@gmail.com

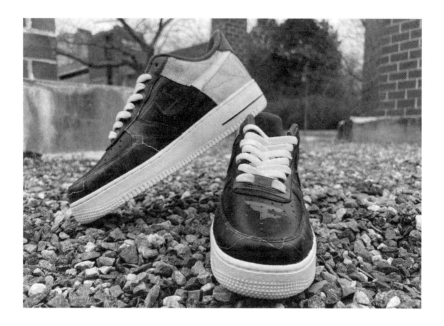

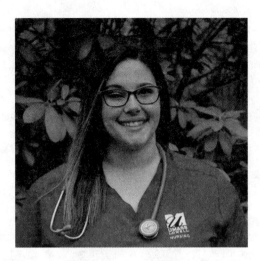

Miranda Melo

"We had the National Guard come in and test the entire facility. So, as a new grad, I was basically put on as a point person for that operation. I was familiar with where the patients were located and their identifiers, so I was sending the troops from the National Guard into each room and directing, making sure that everyone was getting tested and everything was labeled properly."

Miranda is a twenty-two-year-old Registered Nurse who is a first-generation American. Both of her parents were born in the Azores, and she is fluent in Portuguese. In this interview, she talks about her experiences being a recent graduate of UMass Lowell, working in a nursing home at the start of the pandemic and then later at Lowell Community Health Center, and some positive aspects of the lockdown such as redecorating her backyard and spending more time with family.

Miranda Melo was interviewed by Samantha DeMonico on November 15, 2020.

How did your life change during the current Covid-19 pandemic?

So, my life due to Covid was basically flipped upside down. I recently graduated from UMass Lowell in December 2019, from the nursing program. I passed my nursing boards in February. I was hired at Lowell Community Health Center as a new grad, and my job offer was rescinded two days before I was supposed to start. So that definitely threw a curveball in my plans.

I was a little discouraged being a new grad and already losing my first job offer. Thankfully, my mom is a director of nurses at a nursing home in Wakefield, and she agreed to take me on to work over there as a floor nurse and just provide basic care to patients: doing assessments, giving medications, etc. So, that was good. At least it got me a position and I could start working and using my degree. But about two to three weeks into that job we noticed things were definitely changing for the worst. We had patients getting really sick out of nowhere. We had patients passing away at really high rates and that was completely unexpected. So, at that point we kind of realized that there was something a little bit more serious going on, so we decided to test the facility. We found out that about fifteen out of our thirty-four beds were Covid positive. So, really quickly we switched from just a regular unit to a Covid unit and were put in isolation. We had to implement all Covid precautions, and we had the Massachusetts Department of Public Health calling and giving new guideline regulations every day. Everything just moved at a really fast pace as a new grad. It was overwhelming to not only get comfortable with the position but also with all these changes. Learning about the virus each day was just a lot to handle, to say the least.

Is there a particular story you'd like to share about something you've experienced?

The most interesting thing that happened was we had the National Guard come in and test the entire facility. So, as a new grad, I was basically put on as a point person for that operation.

I was really familiar with where the patients were located and their identifiers, so I was sending the troops from the National Guard into each room and directing, making sure that everyone was getting tested and everything was labeled properly. So, it was kind of crazy to be a brand-new grad only working for a few weeks at that point, and basically running an entire Covid testing operation through the entire facility.

What is the typical day like for you now as compared to before the pandemic?

So, I've actually been re-offered the position at Lowell Community Health Center. At the end of June, I was given that position back, so I did start working there. Now, I work full-time at Lowell Community on the adult medicine floor. So, it's definitely a different role that I have now than what I did in the nursing home, because at the nursing home, obviously, the patients are fully dependent. A lot of patient care.

Now, I'm doing primary care so I'm seeing a lot of patients coming in with different symptoms, people calling and saying that they've had exposures to Covid and we have to kind of figure out how high risk they are and what plan of care they should have, whether they should be isolated, quarantined, when they need to get tested, if they need to get retested. And basically, just going about making sure that everybody's staying safe in the community, which like I said is completely different from what I was doing in the nursing home setting.

So what has been most challenging since the lockdown started?

I think the most challenging thing since lockdown has started is that since I've had this new career and these new jobs that I've started throughout the pandemic, I've never really had a way to resume normalcy outside of work. So, it's kind of overwhelming. It's basically getting up in the morning, going to work, getting out of work, and going home every single day. There's not a lot that you can do outside of that at this point, given everything was closed and is now starting to close again.

So, I've lost a lot of the social life aspect of coming out of college and going into this kind of lockdown situation. And it's like, easy to get down on yourself because you feel like all you have to do is get up, go to work, come home, get up, go to work, come home. And it sounds like there's no reward for what you're doing, you know? Yeah, you can't really go out and celebrate, you can't hang out with friends. So, it's easy to get really overwhelmed and down.

Stress levels have increased during the pandemic. What did you do to cope with this?

I would say my stress level has absolutely increased. Not only being a new grad, obviously coming into a new profession is stressful in and of itself. But then, with the constant changing it was super stressful, and not being able to really go anywhere and do anything as a stress outlet, I actually found myself cleaning obsessively. I've literally cleaned my house over and over again, and spent most of the summer, because most things were closed, remodeling my backyard because that was the only place that we could be that was safe, basically. So, we ended up remodeling our entire backyard, making it like a nice patio space so that we could all hang out and be safe and enjoy our time together with the people that live within our own house. So, I spent a lot of time in the backyard hanging out over the summer, and now that it's getting cold, I'm still trying to do bonfires to keep warm, but basically just busy work around the house, trying to not sit in front of the TV for hours and hours and eat food. Yeah, so basically just busy work, a lot of cleaning, a lot of reorganizing.

Are there any positive aspects to life during the pandemic?

I would say yes, because I had a lot more time to spend with my family where during college, I was so busy with school and work. I worked two jobs while I was in my undergrad program that I never really like sat down and had conversations with my parents or with my grandmother who lives with me. Never had a lot of time to just kind of bond and just be with them. Now, since being with anybody else is kind of frowned upon at this point, I've gotten a lot closer with my immediate family than what I would have without the pandemic, which is a nice aspect I find.

Have you reached out for help if you needed it, such as a medical professional, mental health profession, or have you tried to handle it on your own?

I don't think that I've reached a point where I would need to seek out extra help from what I've been able to deal with. I have my mom who's also a nurse, so that kind of helps to be able to go back and forth with stressors and when I need advice. But I would definitely not be against going out to seek help if I found that I was in a position where I need some extra support.

What are your thoughts about mask-wearing?

From a medical standpoint, mask wearing is so unbelievably important. People who don't believe in the power of masking up I feel are just uneducated on the health care repercussions that come with not wearing a mask. And I get that some people say that they can't breathe with it or they have difficulty. But in actuality, putting on a mask can save you and so many other people from becoming sick and possibly having complications of Covid that they pass away or they have long term debilitation from it. Wearing a mask is such a small thing you can do that can cause such a great help in the community. So, I feel like I really push everybody that I know and am close with to wear a mask if possible, and especially socially distance.

Did you take the Covid test? If so, how did that go?

So I've actually been tested, I want to say about eight or nine times so far. When I was working in the nursing home, we were required to get tested pretty frequently just to make sure that we weren't positive and passing it on to other patients. Thankfully, I tested negative each time, which has been a godsend. I also got tested a couple more times because I've had exposures with positive people in the community, including some family members that I've been in contact with that we found out were positive after we had spent two to three days together. I've had a couple of close calls in terms of Covid scares, but thankfully have been able to remain safe and healthy thus far.

What do you think the city of Lowell, and the federal government, can or should do to help keep residents safe and healthy during the pandemic?

One thing I think that should be brought back is at the beginning of the pandemic when Lowell was identified as a hotspot or a red zone, we actually had a program called "Stop the Spread" that is given through the city and the state of Massachusetts. And there was a point throughout the summer where we actually dropped down to I think a yellow or even a green city, so they pulled away our funding for "Stop the Spread" and it was moved to Lawrence because Lawrence was a higher hotspot than we were. I found that's actually a huge disservice to the city of Lowell because there are so many positive cases in Lowell. There are also people who are positive and don't know that they're positive because they don't have access to testing. If you go through urgent care and you don't have symptoms, you do have to pay out of pocket, which a lot of people can't afford. People who don't have insurance don't have primary care so they can't request testing through their primary, either. So, I think it really puts a damper on the ability to be tested adequately.

Thank you for your time and sharing your experiences.

No problem. Thanks for reaching out.

***

Update

 I am now working as the nurse manager of my department at Lowell Community. I am currently coaching a team of elementary school cheerleaders. I have taken some time for myself over the past few years which includes a weight loss journey. In just over one year, I've lost just under eighty pounds by healthy eating and exercising and enjoy sharing my story with my patients as a method of encouragement and health promotion.
—Miranda Melo

3.

Lawrence Community Diary, COVID-19 Pandemic, 2020

4-16-2020

Every day I constantly worry about my parents' health from them working long hours. They need to work to support our family. I know they're scared for their health but they sacrifice themselves since their job is important to build machines for hospitals. I look up to them, they do so much and I don't really get to show them my appreciation. Since there's a pandemic, my parents are Cambodian, they get stared at in stores, they get uncomfortable because they know they aren't sick. People discriminate against Asians because of Covid-19, that's sad to think that a virus can immediately change a view of a race.
—Amanda O., Lawrence, Mass., seventeen years old

4-27-2020

En estos días difíciles durante esta pandemia, mis experiencias no han sido las mejores que murió mi padre allí en la República Dominicana. No pude ir ni despedirme porque los vuelos están suspendidos debido a esta situación, pero aun así trato de compartir con mis otros familiares. También lo amo, pregúntele a todas las personas que si no es necesario salir de la casa, no se vayan, porque así evitaremos reunirnos con otras personas y, de ser así, esta pandemia no se extenderá más, por eso se ocupa de ustedes como así como las otras personas que nos rodean.

Translation: On these difficult days during this pandemic, my experiences have not been the best [since] my father died there in the Dominican Republic. I could not go [there] or say goodbye because the flights [were] suspended due to this situation, but I still try to [keep in touch] with my other relatives. I love [them] too, [and I beg] everyone that, if it is not necessary to leave the house, [to] not leave, because this way we will avoid meeting other people and, if so, this pandemic will not spread anymore. That's [how] it [takes over] you as well as the other

people around us.
—Marlin M., Lawrence, Mass., seventeen years old

5-4-2020

A Brokenhearted Supermarket
As we pull up to our local Stop & Shop, I see a vacant parking lot, with three to four cars, at most. Cautious of our surroundings, we proceed to the entrance. The automatic doors open wide, and a mysterious, eerie breeze hits my face ever so lightly. I stop and stare at the barren shelves and the evident paranoia on every customer's face. I mumble to my mom, "This looks like a scene from a movie!" She sarcastically replies, "So it may be."

A once familiar, family-friendly place had transformed in front of my disoriented eyes. At a quicker than usual pace, we make our way over to the dairy section, stocking up on milk, cheese, and butter before it runs out again. My younger brother reluctantly stretches his skinny arm to the back of the fridge, grabbing the last few cartons of two percent milk. As we complete our "in preparation of a town lockdown" shopping spree and near the self-checkout line, I notice that all toilet paper, hand sanitizer, and soap have gone extinct. It is my first, and hopefully, last, pandemic to live through, so the arrogant behavior of others seems reasonable. I could not help but laugh at how quickly toilet paper became symbolic of the coronavirus crisis. I begin to help my mom bag our groceries when, within the range of my peripheral vision, I see an elder in the check-out line next to ours. The worried man was wearing a tight medical-blue face mask over his nose and mouth. Even though it may have been a cautious procedure, I got sudden butterflies, a haunted fluttery sort of feeling that swept through my stomach. We exit the supermarket, walking six feet behind the person in front of us, looking down at the shiny tiles, wishing that life would return to sanity.
—Hannah G., Andover, Mass., seventeen years old

6-5-2020

I'm feeling a bit conflicted regarding this coming Sunday's Black Lives Matter event on the Common (2 p.m. to 4 p.m.). Part of me wants to attend, pandemic be damned, because I believe we do need change. The other part of me is feeling like I shouldn't go because of the pandemic and I really don't want to get Covid 19 and am afraid that having lots of people gather on the Common will cause it to spread and we'll have a large spike. Also, my mom (seventy-nine years old) and I are planning a weekend away, and I really don't want to get her sick.
—Laura C., Lawrence, Mass., 55 years old

10-15-2020

It has been about a month that school has been in session since shutting down in March due to the pandemic. As a non-teaching member of a school it has been amazing to see all the students, staff, and faculty follow all of the new procedures and safety measures put in place so that we could have students return to the building for some of their learning. Each day I am thankful that we are healthy and happy!

Over the summer I worked on things I never in a million years thought I would:

· I spent a lot of time outdoors, enjoying nature, finding new spots to visit which were off the beaten path.
· I've sewn over two hundred facemasks for friends, family, members of the community (first responders, medical professionals, etc.).
· I spent time noticing best practices of businesses who were promoting social distancing and practicing safety measures and what we could implement at our school.
· I was involved ordering and placing decals throughout the school to remind students to wash hands, wear face masks, etc.

I do look forward to being able to gather safely in large groups, especially at the school I work at. We have shown many ways on how we can come together as a school community virtually, but I do look forward to doing it in person!

—Jessica M., Methuen, Mass., forty-six years old

10-15-2020

Friday, March 13, 2020, was the day everything changed. Seven months later and I can still remember everything that happened that day. No one really took the coronavirus seriously until rumors were starting that school would be closed for the next two weeks. Everyone was excited because we'd get two weeks off and it wasn't that serious yet. In school that day they changed our schedule so we would go to all seven classes instead of five and we would practice zooming with our teachers so when we would be remote we would know what to do. At the end of the day it was insane. Everyone was at their lockers just putting as much as they could into our backpacks because teachers told us to bring everything home just in case. We were told we'd be out of school for a week, and then Governor Charlie Baker would say in a press conference that we'd be closed for longer. I went from everyday driving into Lawrence so I could go to Central Catholic High School to never leaving my house in Methuen. In June, when I had to go pick up my belongings from school, everything seemed different. No one was walking through the parking lot or on the streets, and none of the stores were open. It was like Lawrence had gone from a very busy city to a ghost town.

—Hannah V., Methuen, Mass., seventeen years old

10-15-2020

Covid-19 has our entire school wearing masks to prevent us from getting sick. We have to stay six feet apart at lunch to minimize contact with one another. It's really quite annoying. Luckily no one at our school has it, but the president recently recovered from it so it makes me wonder how bad the virus really is.

—Jack B, Lawrence, Mass., seventeen years old

10-5-2020

This year has been a wild one. I am a senior at Central Catholic High School. Virtual school allowed me to work full time at my job. I work at the Market Basket on Haverhill Street in Methuen as an assistant manager. My parents work long hard hours to have enough money to pay tuition for me and my sister. My dad works as a receiving manager at Gemline, and my mom works at home health VNA. Due to Covid-19, my parents were denied overtime, and my dad was out of work for about two months. I was doing my part in the family by giving my family more than half my paycheck to get us by.

School has been hard—trying to balance the application process and all the assignments my teachers give me with work and family. I'm applying to colleges that I didn't have the chance to visit due to Covid. All my assignments have been online. It's been difficult to adjust.

—Ryan R., Lawrence, Mass., seventeen years old

10-15-2020

The pandemic caused a lot of stress for me personally. It took away something I have loved for my whole life. I could not play baseball and have my junior season at Central Catholic. The effort I put into become more athletic and more versatile was just gone. During quarantine, I had no motivation. I let my body just do whatever it wanted. I gained weight and did not care until we could actually step outside and enjoy being alive. My entire family became sick, and mentally I was not there. I was worried. Many lives were taken, and I was not ready to see my family go if it became worse in my household. Thankfully, my family only became mildly sick and the virus never caused long-term damage or hurt for us. Our bond as a family became stronger, and we were able to conquer our battle with this disease and overcome an obstacle others did not.

—Zariel O., Lawrence, Mass., eighteen years old

11-19-2020

This quarantine is killing me slowly. As each day passes by I feel the motivation to do less and less. All I really want to do at this point is collapse face first into my bed and let the world pass by. Who cares about anything anymore? I just feel so numb to it at this point. So many people are dying and are just in such horrible pain, I'm honestly a bit scared that I might get it, too, especially since I go to school in person with a bunch of other people who refuse to wear masks or just take them off randomly because it's nearly impossible to breathe with the damn things on. The masks are annoying. You can't do anything with friends anymore, and everyone has to be so cautious. I hate this and can't wait for it to be over honestly.

—David G., Lawrence, Mass., fourteen years old

4.

Family, Work, and Community

Sara Morin
Secretary of Lawrence History Center Board of Directors, works for Greater Lawrence Community Action Council

Anábriela Surillo-Navarro
UMass Lowell student, Chuck E. Cheese manager

William Chan
UMass Lowell student, CVS pharmacy technician

Jessica Wilson
Executive Director, Mill City Grows in Lowell

Charlotte,
thank you for
taking the time
to hear us
speak and head
my Story!
— Sara Morin Bartlett

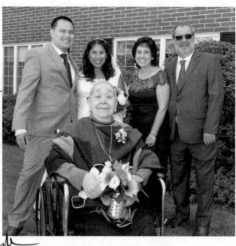

Sara Morin

"People have been incredibly kind, incredibly generous, and it's making me feel hopeful that there are still good things happening in this world, and we don't have to look too far for it either."

Sara Morin was born in Guatemala City, Guatemala, before being adopted and immigrating to Methuen, Mass. She is a Harvard graduate in Museum Studies and the Secretary of the Lawrence History Center Board of Directors, as well as working for Greater Lawrence Community Action Council.

Sara Morin was interviewed by Phillips Academy Spanish language instructor Mark Cutler on May 27, 2020.

Hi, my name is Sara Morin and my pronouns are she, her. My date of birth is February 8, 1988. I was born in Guatemala City, Guatemala, and my hometown now is Methuen, Mass. I currently work for the Greater Lawrence Community Action Council in Lawrence, Mass.

Can you just expand a little bit more on where you are from and how did you initially come to Lawrence?

Yep. So like I mentioned I was born in Guatemala City, Guatemala and my parents adopted me when I was eight months old. I was raised in Methuen, but I was lucky enough to spend time with my grandparents and great grandmother in Lawrence up to around the age of nine. I spent a lot of my time there with my multi-generational family. I had my great-grandmother who was in her late 80s to early 90s and then I had my grandparents as well, and I grew up, and my first second language was Italian because that was the only way I could actually speak with her. And every day my grandfather would walk me down the court and around the corner. So I spent a lot of time in Lawrence when I was very little. It's a comfort place for me because I always think of these really good memories with my family there.

How do you feel now about your home and where you are now?

When it comes to this pandemic, I've thought a lot about what's gone on in history. My great- grandmother came here in 1916; she survived the flu pandemic of 1918. She worked in the mills. She obviously didn't have the technology, didn't have the medicine, didn't have the supplies that we have. So for her to live to be in her nineties with the flu pandemic of 1918 and then all the other things that happened in history, it just reminds me that resiliency exists and that people are strong, and there's a lot to be hopeful for. So I think in terms of this pandemic, it's given me a lot to think about. There's a lot to reflect on, and when I thought about doing this oral history it was kind of nice to think through the albums and look through my family's history and just remind myself that we've been through a lot, and we're gonna get through this, and I think things are gonna be okay.

How are you maintaining your relationship with your grandmother and your connection to your roots and family through all of this?

It's been interesting. Two weeks ago, I finally got to see her for the very first time, and when I say see, it means looking at my grandmother through a glass door. But it made a world of difference mentally for me because to see that she's ninety-three years old and was happy as a clam to see us, and to know that she's safe during this pandemic definitely makes things a lot easier.

Every time I talk to her, she always has three things to say: the first is I have no regrets, the second is I'm not afraid, and the third is she reminds me to keep on kicking. So it's nice to know that she's pretty resilient. I always remind my family, too, that my grandmother was one of the smallest babies born during her time in 1927. She was born on Taylor Street in Methuen, but when she was born she was I think one pound, like she was a tiny preemie, and she always told me that when she came home from the hospital they put her by the fireplace and they had to keep the bassinet there and were really worried. So when I think of my grandmother I always think of strength because she started off as this tiny preemie in 1927 and she's ninety-three, and she's lived through the pandemic. She remembers Pearl Harbor. She remembers, you know, Kennedy. She remembers all of these different historical points in her life. She survived 9/11, so I would say she's like my rock right now, so anytime she says keep on kicking it reminds me—okay, like keep on living, keep on going.

Can you tell us a little bit more about how you've integrated yourself in the community? What is it that you're doing in the community?

Right now, the one thing that's keeping me going is knowing that my job is helping people in the community. I started at the Greater Lawrence Community Action Council in 2019. My job, like any job in the museum field or any other job, you tend to wear many hats. I am the development associate, but right now I am on outreach duty where I'm reaching out to different vendors, different businesses, which is very difficult right now, to see if we can get donations for our food pantry. Every Tuesday we have a food pantry from 4:30 p.m. to 5:30 p.m., and before the pandemic we were helping close to 100 families and individuals who would come to get extra food just for the week. We were lucky enough to get grants that allow us to have refrigeration and freezer capabilities, that way we can get food that is obviously just a little bit more than a can of beans and a bag of rice, which is pretty awesome. So as of right now, I think, last week we hit 340 families and individuals. So obviously with this pandemic the need is incredibly great to help people, our neighbors, that's really what it is—it's helping our neighbors and our loved ones, and the one thing that keeps me going is knowing that what I'm doing right now is making a difference. It may not seem very big, but knowing that I maybe got an extra box of beans or was able to track down some masks for people waiting in line, or starting a food drive in Methuen, which is kind of nice, it can bridge the communities of Greater Lawrence a little bit. It helps remind me that there are good things happening and it makes me feel hopeful.

What else is the Greater Lawrence Community Action Council doing for the people of Lawrence and the community?

On top of the food pantry we are still enrolling people in need for fuel assistance. It sounds kind of crazy given today at nine o'clock it was sixty-eight degrees! It's starting to feel like summer, but people have bills to pay. And some people that I've talked to have close to over a thousand dollars' worth of bills with home heating, and they need help. When the pandemic started rolling back in March we still needed heat, and a lot of these people have families, a lot of them live alone, so who's going to help them? Especially if they're out of work or unfortunately, a lot of the elderly people don't have families the way we think of, you know, sometimes it's just one person. So they obviously need help. We allow home visits as long as it's safe to make sure that these people are getting not only social interaction, but the help that they need. We also have our WIC (Women, Infants & Children) office, and right now the critical need for them are diapers, wipes, and formula. So a lot of these people are out of jobs and the unemployment rate is pretty high right now. If you're lucky enough to be able to keep your job you can kind of balance things out a little bit with your life, but if you're sick with Covid-19 you can't go to work, your family's quarantined for two weeks, so a lot of these people can't even leave their house. So then they reach out to us and we do the best that we can to do drop-offs on their porch and make sure that they're well taken care of in the best way that we can.

Is the Greater Lawrence Community Action Council looking for volunteers?

We're always looking for volunteers to help us. With the food pantry especially, we could always use people packing the bags, and then obviously for distribution where we have close to 400 people now waiting in line. It's helpful to have people make sure everyone keeps their six feet social distancing so everyone kind of feels safe. It would be great to have more people mobilize units where we can do more drop-offs. We do know we have a large amount of clients who are unable to come down to the food pantry, so I'm crossing my fingers that maybe if we build up enough volunteers that we can start mobilizing people to do more drop-offs. Any help that we can get we're super appreciative of it, because we know that there's a lot of uncertainty when it comes to being out in public. Right now things seem a little scary in Lawrence because we've ramped up testing, so obviously the number of Covid-19 cases are gonna skyrocket. It's not that we're doing anything wrong, it's just we've been given the testing that we have and it's making people aware of how to stay safe out there. So there is a little bit of uncertainty with people coming in to volunteer, they're a little skeptical, but it's just reminding people to be safe and follow best practices—wash your hands, wear a mask, stay six feet apart. We will do our very best to keep all our volunteers and staff safe.

Are you working with anybody else in the city, community to make this work happen? Do you have partners in the city that are also supporting this that you are collaborating with?

So right now the Merrimack Valley Food Bank has been really great about supplying us with food. Things have been a little scarce when it comes to food, but they've always had something for us to pick up, and we're so grateful for that. The mayor has been great when it comes to supporting us once he realized that we had so many people coming to our food pantry because they felt safe. We really, really emphasized the six feet apart rule. We have lines on the sidewalk and that wraps all the way down Essex Street, all the way up towards the bus station, all the way towards Buckley Transportation Center and around, almost back around the block. So he's been really great about providing some form of police presence, not because things are unruly, but just to make sure that everything stays organized. And if something should happen there's someone there to protect the people and the staff and volunteers. Everyone's been really great support-ing us. The Senior Center knows what we're doing and they're constantly re-posting everything that we're posting, so I mean if anyone gets referred to us, it's always because either word of mouth or because someone was genuinely generous enough to recommend us to somebody from the community.

What has the Covid 19 pandemic meant to you—what have you changed or what has been impacted?

I stopped working physically at work, I want to say March 15th, I think that was the day. I have to actually go into work at some point and look at the date on the calendar there, because I have one of those flip calendars and I'm kind of attributing that day is when the world just kind of shifted on me. So I stopped physically working in the office on one of those days during the week of St. Patrick's Day, and it's been interesting. My mom works at the very nursing home that my grandmother is at, so my grandmother is holding on pretty good right now because of that. She's comforted knowing that there's somebody in the building who is there for her. Even though my mom can't see her for safety reasons, just knowing someone's in the next room over is a little bit comforting. So it's been a little scary because my mom is taking people's temperatures and she's right on the front lines when people walk in, and I've kind of been holding my breath a little bit with that, but knock on wood she got her Covid test and tested negative. So did my grandmother when the National Guard came in to test everyone there a few weeks back.

But I guess for me, I didn't realize how much you missed things until they're gone. So I've really been in tune with my mental health when it came to this pandemic. When this first started, I was actually getting panic attacks before, during, and after leaving the market and I never had that happen before. Even wearing a mask, I don't know, it was just very odd to me, and having people wait in line just made it seem all the more overwhelming. It took a while for me to finally feel like, Okay, this is the new norm, I have to accept this and this is how it's going to be. During the peak in April, I think, it was the 10th of April to the 20th of April where the governor said, "If you don't have to be out, don't go out." We've really tried very hard not to go out anywhere. And now I'm at that point where I can walk into the market wearing my mask, and I use my hand sanitizer, and I don't get that pain in my chest when it comes to going to the market anymore. I think that's because I've just accepted that this is the way life is now. But for a while there taking me to the market was like a whole other experience. I cried and I just felt so overwhelmed by everything, but I think things are gonna be okay. On top of this, I'm trying really hard to be happy about planning a wedding in September, and that's also been a little bit of a challenge sometimes because up until this point I haven't felt very hopeful about having a wedding. And I've actually come up with a "plan b" where my parents have graciously offered having ten people in their backyard and will get a little tent and the Justice of the Peace said, "I'll still come and I'll marry you guys." For me that's really important, because the day that we picked is September 20th, 2020. We really love that date, and then we came to the realization that it also was my great-grandfather's birthday—he would have been 100 years old that day. So it had even more meaning for us. I think regardless of what happens, we're gonna get married that day because life doesn't stop for Covid, it doesn't stop for illnesses, it doesn't stop for anything. Even if we have to wear a mask, we will. But it's definitely been a roller coaster—you have your good days, you have your bad days, and it's trying to find the little joys in life.

So I think you said you were quarantining with your mother and your father.

That's right.

How about your fiancé, where does he come into the picture?

So we've been really good about creating almost like a little vacuum when it comes to being around other individuals. If I'm not here at my house with my parents, I'm in Methuen with my fiancé and his brother. Other than that, those are the only people that I see. I won't obviously visit friends. It's just a matter of creating this vacuum where we can trace where we've been, that way if something should happen it'll be a little bit easier. You know we've only gone to the market when we have to, and it's been nice in a way to have another place to visit, because my dad's been around my fiancé and his brother. So, you know, if he wants he can go over there and play cards, because right now his brother is out of work because he works in the hospitality business, and my fiancé actually just started a new job yesterday. Surprisingly enough he was able to find another job and, knock on wood it lasts because obviously the unemployment rates are really high right now, so we're feeling very blessed and grateful for that.

Had he been out of work until he found this job, and is this because of the pandemic that he was out of work?

He worked for a small business accounting firm and with every-thing going on, in his mind, it was more of, if small businesses are starting to cut back on things, one of the first things they'll cut back on is a luxury accounting service that'll do everything for them, because you have to cut your costs to make sure that you can still stay in business. So he had just been looking and thankfully came across another company and they said, "Yeah, we need someone right now, this is our busy time because of the pandemic." They're a health care supplies place so they need help.

Is there anything that you're doing currently that you think you might continue doing when the pandemic subsides?

One of the things that I've found that has been extremely help-ful—and thankfully the weather's been great for this—is walk-ing. My mom and I had the habit of going to the gym every morn-ing and walking on the treadmills for a little bit even before our day started, and when the pandemic broke out it was still pretty chilly so that we really couldn't walk out too too much, but once it started ramping up it was probably about April and we were like, we need to walk, we need to keep moving, we need to like keep helping us help ourselves. So I think walking will definitely be one of those things. We went for a walk this morning and it was sixty-eight degrees out, but we still got our walk in because it mentally made us feel good. It's been a new routine for us and I think that's one of those things that definitely has to stick.

What are things that you hold onto that give you hope in life, both in general and during the pandemic?

Well, like I said my mantra right now is just keep on kicking, it's something my grandmother always said and it's holding kinda true right now, just keep on kicking, just keep moving, just keep living, like just keep going. I guess I've been feeling more hopeful lately with everything going on. I think that's, like I said, because I've just adjusted, and finally I feel like one day the light bulb went on and everything just clicked into gear and I finally just accepted that this is the way things are. It took a load off my shoulders because I'm finally not stressing out as much as I used to about everything going on.

I think moving forward hope is—for me anyways—looking at how we help each other, and being hopeful that there are still kind, good people out there who are willing to help when the chips are down. I always think of the Mr. Rogers quote where he said, "Look for the helpers when things are bad." It's me paraphrasing it, but you know even when 9/11 happened my mom always told me look for the good things, and I think that's where I'm at right now. I'm just looking for all the good that's happening from this. I recently came across some cloth masks, or actually just some cloth and I reached out to a local community group, and I said, "Hey help me out, I have this cloth, I have the thread, but I don't have the sewing machine, it's going to take me like four hours just to sew one mask, is anyone able to help me?" And people popped right up and said, "Yeah just drop off the cloth, drop off the thread, and I'll be so happy to help you," and you know I asked for six masks and I got twelve.

So people have been incredibly kind, incredibly generous, and it's making me feel hopeful that there are still good things happening in this world. And we don't have to look too far for it either, because every time I go [to the food pantry] on a Tuesday, as heartbreaking as it is to see that line grow each week, it makes me feel good and hopeful that we're still able to do what we do. And if that means just giving someone an extra meal that means keeping someone hungry one less day. I know that when this whole thing is over I'm still gonna look for that hope. You know, don't overlook it when things get bad and just keep looking for it because it's there.

Is there anything that I haven't brought up or that you haven't mentioned that you'd like to offer right now?

One of the things that I think Lawrence is struggling with right now is the fact that a lot of the celebrations that we have are not going to happen this year. Semana Hispana, the Bread and Roses Heritage Festival, the Feast of the Three Saints, the Mahrajan, all those things that we think of, you know Semana Hispana usually kicks off summer—and I think it's one of those things that we have to remind ourselves that even if they're not happening or they're not happening in the conventional way that we think of, that we can still celebrate those festivals in our own way. I was digging through some of my pictures and I was thinking, like especially where my family is Sicilian, we always think of the Feast. You know we just have to keep going and we can still celebrate these events in our own way. It was so nice to see that the Bread and Roses Heritage Festival is gonna do this virtually, so we're still gonna have it, it's just a matter of finding new and innovative ways to celebrate the things that we want, and the things that are important to us. So it's nice to see that we're still gonna move forward, and Lawrence is going to become innovative with their ways of doing all of these things.

***

Update

Since the interview, a lot has changed in my life. I did get married on September 20, 2020. Despite her being in the nursing home, I was able to see and hug my grandmother on my wedding day and I cherish the pictures I have from that day. My grandmother passed away in October 2021. I changed jobs in December 2021. I am now the Associate Director of Development at Esperanza Academy in Lawrence, Massachusetts. I am grateful to have the opportunity to continue to work in the Lawrence community and be in a place that holds such wonderful memories for me—Sara Morin Barth*

*Note: After her marriage, Sara Morin's name changed to Sara Morin Barth.

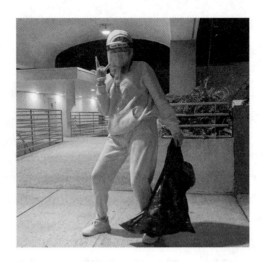

Anábriela Surillo-Navarro

"When I arrived [in Puerto Rico], the hug that my mom gave me was like this [air hug]. She didn't want to touch me, you know, and I get it. And I understand what's happening. So, like, the next morning, I went and got tested, I got negative, I didn't have it. So that's when my mom gives me a hug."

Anábriela Surillo-Navarro is a twenty-three-year-old resident of New Hampshire, working as a general manager for Chuck E. Cheese in Lowell and also finishing her bachelor's degree at UMass Lowell. She describes her ethnicity as Puerto Rican, having moved to the States from the island at the age of twenty. In this interview, Anábriela discusses difficulties in the workplace, living away from her family, and her concerns about the virus.

Anábriela was interviewed by Nejaray Torres on November 5, 2020.

So how has your life changed during the current Covid-19 pandemic?

I think we're always afraid. I mean, myself and my boyfriend Esteban, we're here alone, like our whole family, his mom, his sister, his niece, and all of mine are in Puerto Rico. So, if we actually get Covid very, very bad which he had, I didn't. It was rough, you know, thinking of what if he dies? What if this goes to another extent that I can't help him? Or what if it impacts me?

We traveled three months ago to Puerto Rico. And I remember, when I arrived, I went all covered up. It's four hours from here to Puerto Rico, so I wore a haircap, I wore my face mask, my shield. I think I have a picture. There was no possibility that I could, like, you know, get in contact with it. But still, obviously, my job here, I never stopped working . . . well for two weeks I did, but when I arrived there, the hug that my mom gave me was like this [air hug]. She didn't want to touch me, you know, and I get it. And I understand what's happening. So, like, the next morning, I went and got tested, I got negative, I didn't have it. So that's when my mom gives me a hug. So, obviously I respect that because she is fifty-five years old. If it hits me, it's not going to be the same as if it hits her. When it comes to how have our lives changed, and I think we're always, always the people that are aware that this is a serious issue. We're very on the lookout, like, Oh, no, I don't want to do this. My friends, both of them got it a month ago, I haven't seen them. And they showed me a paper that says negative. They got it last week.

But you're still scared?

I still will not see them. It's not because I stopped loving them or it means anything related to the affection I have towards them, but mostly because I want to keep myself good. Meaning that if I get kicked out of work, like let's say I have to quarantine, what's going to pay my bills? You feel me?

Exactly. Yeah. That's good that you've had a job throughout the whole thing. Is there a particular story you'd like to share about something you experienced?

Um, he's [Esteban] not going to like this one. He got it. He got it at the beginning, but his was very mild. I think I never got it because when I came back from Puerto Rico, I did both of the tests. I got negative in the nasal and I got negative in the blood, meaning that mostly, I didn't have it. Again, I don't know how that works, I'm not a chemist.

He's very young. How I say this? Like you push him and he's "Oh, it hurts." So, I think that the only funny thing that happened was that I had to care for him in ways like you know, soup here, soup there. Massage here, pills here, like he wouldn't be able to do stuff. And I get it. I mean, it hits differently, but I don't think how it hit him was very like, rough. He had head-aches and whatever. But what I could see, it wasn't like "Oh I can't do nothing." Same for my friends. I call my friends, I FaceTime my friends all the time and they got it, but it wasn't rough versus other people that have told me it has been like a big thing. A serious thing.

What is the typical day like for you now as compared to before the pandemic?

First of all, I always forget my mask. I get very annoyed every time I have to go back to the car to look for my mask. We've been what, six, seven months on this I thought that by now I'll be like, Okay, it's part of the routine. As I grab my phone, I get my mask, but it hasn't happened like that. And I think we're always very skeptical about who we come into contact with. For me, like balancing my life, meaning obviously, for me school's first, but work obviously will be second. But my social life is there too, you know. I'd rather just not go out, like here in New Hamp-shire clubs are open. I'm not going to go to clubs, there's no way you're going to find me in a club. No. So when it comes to how life has changed in my daily basis, I think we're more aware this is a natural thing, it's killing tons of people. Oh, very paranoid in the fact that I have hand sanitizer everywhere. And like, Oh, let me clean my hands here. Or when I go to the gas station, I put gloves on, I have gloves in my car. In terms of things that I cannot control, I cannot clean beforehand, I'm very paranoid. But things that I can control, for example, my house and whatever, I will say it is Covid-free because no one comes inside except us. But again, I'll do what I can, you know. Covid is a thing that you can get multiple times. Let's say at first you get it like, Oh, I lost the taste or the smell. That's nothing or whatever, but you don't want to get it a second time because you don't know if the second time, you're going to be this lucky.

Exactly. That's crazy. I was wondering that. I was like, Can you get it more than once? And you just answered my question.

Yes. I mean, that's what I have read that you can because, even if you have immunity, when the second wave hits, let's say you were not drinking your vitamins or whatever, and then for any reason you've gotten in contact with someone or multiple people. You never know.

What has been most challenging during the pandemic?

So when the pandemic hit, Chuck E. Cheese got very hit, a lot of stores closed. We filed for bankruptcy, we thought we were going to lose our jobs. We were fourteen stores in my district, from those fourteen stores, four closed and we got transferred too, so now we're twelve. We thought the slow profit stores were the ones that were going to close. So, at one point, I was very nervous because one of the lowest impacts when it comes to profit, it's Lowell's store. So, I was like, God, I'm going to lose my job. And I thought that was going to happen, you know, I thought okay so Leominster closed, Danvers closed, Natick closed, so we're the next one. Little did I know, phase three started so we were able to open, we were able to make profit, not as we're used to for this month, but still we are making more profit than when we were closed. So, I think that was my biggest worry.

When it came to Esteban and his job, if he had a fever, he wouldn't go to work, he couldn't. It was like that. They were very strict. So that made it rough because obviously he wasn't making enough money. And he's a person that takes care of himself. He doesn't like to go out. All he does is the PlayStation. But still in his job they were very precautious. When it comes to Chuck E. Cheese, just to give you the versus, like yeah, we take temperatures, and we do stuff. There was one day that Esteban apparently came in close contact with someone in his older job that tested positive. And, um, so what happened was that I called my boss and I told them, "Hey, this is what happened." Esteban didn't have anything, like he never presented any symptoms. But he still came in contact. I thought they would tell me, "Hey, take a couple of days" or whatever, which they didn't. Apparently how Human Resources works was just asking how close he was with him and whatever. They asked me a couple of questions, but decided that I didn't have to quarantine, which was okay. I mean, money. [Laughter] But you know when it comes to the jobs he has had, they were very precautious like if you came in close contact with someone in the same unit, they sent the whole unit into quarantine.

Have your stress levels changed during the pandemic?

Oh, look at my face girlfriend [referring to pimples]. Look at my face, you tell me.

What did you do to cope with this?

Oh, nothing. Look at me, look at me. I'm buying pharmacy products. I'm buying that to cure this. I think it's, so two things. And I think you can say the same. First of all, Covid you know, like, having a mask every single time. Inhalando y exhalando [inhaling and exhaling], you understand Spanish?

Yeah.

Inhalando y exhalando in my own face. Makes you get pimples and all that, right? But the fact that, I don't know, professors are thinking that they want to test your commitment in school, right? In one of my classes my professor, she does a pre-class quiz. She gives an assignment every Sunday, and she gives an after-discussion quiz. So, there are three things for the same class. Completely unnecessary. So imagine that with six classes, it's completely stressful, like being able to manage everything. And then I'll start touching my face when I'm doing my projects, and all that. So, I think when it comes to stress, everyone is stressing. They're testing our limits. You know, they're just testing how we react.

So, are there any positive aspects to your life during the pandemic?

Cheap flights? [Laughter] I was able to go to Puerto Rico for less than 170 bucks. Round trip. What else? I don't think anything else; I only think cheap flights was the one. My Christmas tickets—we're going for Christmas and Christmas tickets usually are seven, eight, nine thousand dollars. Or a hundred, not a thousand. And this year, we managed to get it for $500. So, cheap price and you have social distancing when you buy tickets on JetBlue.

Oh, they have social distancing on flights?

They don't. Frontier doesn't even care. They take your temperature. They give you hand sanitizer, whatever, but you sit next to someone. The only airline is JetBlue.

Did you receive help when/if you needed it, like if you needed groceries or someone to go shopping for you, something like that?

So now, I think when the pandemic hit and all that, a lot of franchises made a lot of profit having you know, touchless deliveries. So, Amazon I know made a lot of money, same for supermarkets because they charge you a fee to do this. And I think the help that I got was that instead of me going to Walmart when I knew that there was a lot of people, I could just do a Google search and then order it to come to my house, instead of me exposing myself. You know when it hit in March, everyone was like, "Oh my god, I cannot leave my house." So, I think social media helped us to have a tool to keep getting the stuff that we need but not expose ourselves, kind of.

When it comes to other stuff, I think CVS had a lot of propaganda that they were doing the test. They gave you an immediate response, which was the one Esteban took, and it was positive. That was great because he could know the same day if he had it or not, but then they changed it to seven to ten days. So, I don't respect that one because now you have to wait ten days to know if you actually have it or not. So, in ten days, you're not making money. I know they can because the blood one, it gives you a false positive if you do have it and at least you know okay, so either I had it or I have it. But not being able to have the response quickly, I think that's something they have to work on.

What about mask wearing?

It's necessary, and I hate when people put it here [gestures below the nose]. In Chuck E. Cheese, I have to constantly tell people, "Masks go above your nose." If you just put it here, it's not working. You're not doing anything. And if I can have my face like this [breaking out], because of my mask, I feel like everyone can too. [Laughter] El dióxido de carbono [the carbon dioxide].

It's so annoying, literally.

And it's here, look [pointing to chin with acne]. It's not even, if you tell me, if it's stress it would be here, [pointing to cheeks] but it's literally where you wear the mask.

Do they make you wear a specific mask at Chuck E. Cheese or just any mask is fine?

No, any mask. I bought a couple, like the ones that were like las que están cocidas [those that are sewn]. I bought a couple; I don't know where they are. So, I'm wearing a Chuck E. Cheese brand one.

Do they make you pay? Or they just give them to you?

No, no, they just have us wear a mask. We just take them.

You mentioned that you got two Covid tests already. How did those go?

So, I got three. When I arrived in Puerto Rico, I got the blood test. I have tattoos, but I am afraid of needles, as stupid as it might sound. [Laughter] I know, I know, I know. But it was easy. I do have to say the nurse was really good. I didn't even feel it, so that was okay. I got my results within two hours, even earlier than that. I was so happy because I wanted to hug my grandma, my grandma has been through a lot of things. She was diagnosed with cancer for the third time, and I actually wanted to hug her. So, once I got the results, I went directly to her house and then hugged her.

When I was coming back here, after Puerto Rico, I did the nasal. It didn't hurt, like people will tell me "Oh, that's going to hurt" blah, blah, blah. But where I went, which is in Gurabo [town in Puerto Rico] they did a blood test, which was the same thing. Um, and then when they did the nose one, they told me to put my head up. And then they put the nasal Q-tip or whatever it's called, you know how they put it in and rub it? They didn't rub it. They just put it in and asked me to put my head back like this, and then they left it for ten seconds. And then they told me to keep breathing those ten seconds. Then they took it out, put it here [other nostril] and did the same thing for ten seconds. They just left it there and made me breath, so that way, the particles touch the thing. I was blessed because I didn't have a bad experience. I actually had a good one.

How have things been different for you in terms of self-care and cleaning your house?

Um, cleaning my house? I think the same. I mean, well, cleaning-wise. Cleaning-wise in my house, I think the same, we clean. It's not like it's different. I don't have the sprayer here or the hand sanitizer here. People don't come here. Like I don't, again, we don't have family members here. So, the only people that could come here is his best friend or my friends. And it doesn't happen a lot.

So, if they come and they have it, then I'll be very F'd. Because I didn't do nothing. [Laughter] But in regards to self-care, I have to do it more. I bought the products to be able to do it. But with all the stress, again, with school and work and the mask, and that stress that you always have because you don't know who has it because they can be asymptomatic and then you come in contact with them. I think that stress has made us tired. We're always tired. I could sleep all day, I can sleep ten hours and still be tired and I say it's because of that. Before this, I wasn't, you know, that stressed, but we're always constantly thinking of "Oh, what if I already had it?" Or "What if I got it?" Or "What if this person came to my house and he has it? What's going to happen?"

Right. You have no idea. Exactly. So, last question. What do you think the city of Nashua and/or the federal government can/should do to help keep residents safe and healthy during the pandemic?

Oh, I can talk about both of them. I did live over there in Lowell, and I think Massachusetts is doing a great job. I think the governor is very aware of the cities and very aware of what is happening. I know this because of my work. Now, they have a curfew.

The ways that they are implementing it, I think is giving us the chance to take care of ourselves as we should. I still think they should be stricter. Puerto Rico, it's very strict over there, in terms of they've had a curfew since the beginning of March. They still have a curfew; they've been opening things for you to do and whatnot, but I think that's because of the election to be honest. They're going to go back to how strict they were.

Comparing both, New Hampshire and Massachusetts, I feel like Massachusetts' governor has been more aware that this is an actual problem going on and people are dying versus New Hampshire. I moved here in May, and in July, to say something, already restaurants are open. Already you can dine in, already you can do this and that. The clubs are open; I see people going to clubs without masks and just enjoying life like nothing is happening, which is very alarming. You never know, and not even us, the elderly. You never know if sick people come across me, and I take care of my grandma and I give it to her, and she dies. So, I think New Hampshire in particular is not responsible in terms of taking care of their people versus Massachusetts. Even though we can do more to protect us as citizens, they are trying their best to implement rules for us to follow and stay safe.

There are places like Argentina. When you compare Argentina to the United States, when it comes to money, obviously the United States has a lot more. And Argentina closed completely; no one can go out, no one can come in. Why? Because they want to prevent the spread, if people have it . . . And then, whenever everything clears up, whenever there is a vaccine, then we can reopen. That's just thinking ahead because you don't want all these people to die and sadly, it's not people like us dying. Yeah, there are some cases of course, but the people that are being hit harder are the people whose health is more compromised. It's not the same thing, and I was telling my brother this, going above a hill, it's not the same thing me and my brother walking up the hill than me, my brother, and my grandmother. Half-way up the hill, my grandmother will be out of breath. Why? Because her health is compromised. If it hits her, it's going to hit different. She's going to have more . . . and now that she has cancer, it's even worse because now her immune system is all F'd up, you know?

She's at risk.

And we want to keep it safe for those people. This is what I think New Hampshire does, they're just thinking of their money you know? How we can keep the economy moving, how we can stop the unemployment rate. They stopped giving the money out, and I get it, a lot of people were abusing this, but still . . . .

A lot of people need it, too.

Yeah, what are you going to put first: the money or your people? The people were the ones that chose you, you know?

Exactly.

I think we have to think more of others, meaning the elderly, than us when it comes to topics like health.

Is there anything we didn't discuss that you would like to add?

Nope. I think they were good questions.

Anábriela, thank you so much for taking the time to talk with me today.

Of course.

***

Update

In January 2021, Abuela passed away and this influenced my decision about staying in the United States. Shortly after I graduated from UMass Lowell I decided that home was and will always be, close to my family. I came back to Puerto Rico, where things aligned properly and not only did I find a great general manager position at a park (Altitude Trampoline Park, Bayamon to be exact), I was able to find a decent apartment, lease a car, and find an incredible partner who has helped me step up and move forward. He has a young four-year-old daughter who I adore and life has been awesome. In terms of Covid, down here in the island things were rough, people continue suffering from this virus and the government forced everyone to be vaccinated (three doses up to now) for a while. But recently it changed, and they aren't asking for vaccinations, masks, or even negative test results. So, since March 10, 2022, life is as if Covid never happened here. Lucky for me I do love wearing a mask and I'm constantly cleaning my hands and surroundings—Anábriela Surillo-Navarro

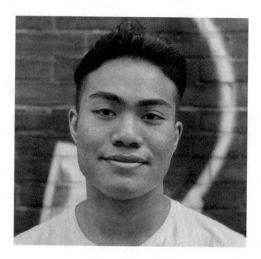

William Chan

"And from my experience, a majority of older Cambodian generations, people that I know, I feel like a lot of people here don't have the ability to work from home . . . You know, that goes for my parents, they can't stay home and work . . . they always have to go in every day to work, of course with masks, but they're so susceptible to gaining the virus that it's unfortunate that they have to go through that."

William is a twenty-one-year-old student at UMass Lowell majoring in Biology and a pharmacy technician at CVS. He has lived in Lowell his entire life with his family. He describes his ethnicity as half Cambodian and half Thai. In this interview, William speaks about difficulties he experienced working at the pharmacy, helping his parents, and how different races, ethnic groups, and socioeconomic classes in Lowell were affected by the pandemic. Towards the end of the interview, William and Jonathan compare their experiences living in Lowell and Reading.

William Chan was interviewed by Jonathan Hohler on October 27, 2020.

We're going to talk about your experiences during the pandemic. How has your life changed during the Covid-19 pandemic?

Well, whenever it first started, it was a huge shift. Typically, I'm a pretty active individual. I am a director and a dancer on a team in Boston. I participate in a lot of clubs at the school [UMass Lowell]. I do a lot of volunteering.

When the pandemic happened, there was so much change where I had to take away all that and just stay home. And typically, I'm so used to being active that staying home, even though I'm introverted, didn't feel right to me. If I felt like I wasn't doing it, I wasn't being productive. I didn't realize how much I used activities to avoid my mental health. So, because of that, everything just crashed down at once. And for a few weeks, it was like one of the worst times of this year for me. But at the same time, it was a blessing in disguise, because I kind of found who I truly am as a person, rather than running away from it

Do you have any particular story you'd like to share about something you experienced?

Like any story, like that I experienced during the pandemic? In the beginning, even though I lost a lot of connection physically with people that I knew, they actually brought a lot of connections I lost back to me, you know, a lot of people talking like, "Hey, how are you doing? Are you okay?" Just people checking up on you. I feel like that made you realize who actually cared and wanted to check in on you, rather than just seeing them in person. Because you can see someone in person, but does it actually mean that they're there for you? Does it actually mean they care about your well-being? So, when you rebuild those connections that you've lost, it kind of brings back another relationship or connection that you never knew you had before. During the pandemic, I think that's a thing that really stood out to me. Because there's a lot of people that didn't think I would ever talk to them again. But now we're closer because of what happened.

What is the typical day for you now as compared to before the pandemic?

During the summer, when there wasn't school every day, it was kind of just wake up, go on YouTube, Netflix, or read. Once I'm bored with that, I go along and drive by myself or I go for a walk by myself, of course, secluded. Or there was one time that I went on a walk with a friend, but we were like, across the street from each other and just talking on the phone, just to be careful. But yeah, typically during the summer, it was just wake up, go to bed. On the weekends, I work at the pharmacy. So, I would go to work. But now during school, wake up, take classes online to stay home, eat. I didn't go to work when I'm scheduled to go to work. I don't really do much.

So, how's that different from before? How has your day to day changed?

So before, obviously, like when we were in person, I would go to classes and I'd stay at school probably until 8 p.m. I typically had classes from the morning all the way to 5 p.m. And then I would use that time to study or just hang out with friends, or on Tuesdays and Thursdays, that's when I would have practice in Boston. So, I go to Boston pretty often, too, and just meet up with friends there or like schedule practices there with my team. I would go to workshops on weekends after work. I did a lot of different activities just to keep myself busy and being active. You know, like how I said, once the pandemic hit, all that was taken away in the blink of an eye. And at that moment, you don't really know what to do because it's so sudden that you didn't really prepare for it. Like no one was prepared for it. So, it's kind of like okay, yeah.

What has been the most challenging about this?

I think the most challenging thing for me was just limiting your-self from seeing people. I guess not being able to physically be with those who you want to be with all the time. I think that's the hardest thing because I'm a person who likes to be around people, regardless if I don't talk that much, because I like the company of people. But because of everything, you can't really do that with just anyone, and you can't make new friendships like that, because you need to be cautious. And, you know, you can't just go to a party, or like, go to a park and be like, "Hi. How are you doing?" Because it's, it's not going to work that way. It's for the safety of us, you know?

Have your stress levels changed during the pandemic?

Yes, in a good way, but in the beginning, in a bad way. So, in the beginning, like I said, because I avoided all the mental stability of myself, it was a lot harder for me. So, it brought on more stress to myself when I didn't need to, because I had to face things I always avoided. But after, especially, like, more recently, now, I've been able to manage that stress well and really look at things in more of a problem-solving way instead of, Oh, this is never going to be fixed. So, now in terms of when I'm stressed, I'm like there's always going be a solution to something and I don't need to be overwhelmed. You know, regardless of if it's school, or it's like a personal thing, because at that moment, it's only going to happen for that moment and it's not going to stay there for a lifetime.

So, you say that you coped with that stress by kind of changing the context?

Yes.

Are there any positive aspects to your life during the pandemic?

Positive?

Anything new, or something that you wouldn't have had before. For example, you talked about, you know, you got a lot of connections from people that you haven't spoken to, which is a good thing so would you say that's a positive change?

I feel like a positive thing was that I've become more comfortable with myself not caring what other people think, because I don't need the opinions of others to validate myself. If I'm happy, I'm happy. And I think that was a really uplifting thing to feel during this time.

Okay, awesome. How did you seek help if and when you needed it?

Because we're so limited on contact with people in person, the best thing you can do is text or call those who are there for you. That's what I did. Honestly, it varies from person to person, but for me, just contacting people—or like talking to my sister because she's the closest person to me—about things that are going on or what advice I should need to use, you know, depending on the situation, because there's not really much you can do, you know.

Have you ever gotten a Covid test?

Yes, I actually got one today.

How did it go?

It went pretty well. So, I went to CVS, because depending on where you're going in Massachusetts, you would have to get referred from a doctor in order for your insurance to cover it. If you don't, if you just go by yourself, you have to pay out of pocket for that. But most CVSs take insurance, and you don't really need a referral from a doctor as long as you pass a list that they give you, some things to check off. But it was pretty easy. I went, I scheduled an appointment at about 11 a.m. It was a self-test, so I did it myself. So, they gave me a bag and in it was a nose swab. I just shoved it up there and it didn't feel too bad to do it. It was for both nostrils and it just feels like a little itch, like you kind of have to hold your sneeze, so you don't sneeze out the cotton swab. But it's about one inch, just shove it up. Hold it for fifteen seconds, put it in a test tube, and then you get it back to them. Pretty easy.

Did you feel it touch your brain, like people are saying?

No, I think people were just exaggerating about that.

How have things been different for you in terms of self-care and things such as cleaning your house?

My family and I definitely try to wipe door handles down, like the most hand-used items in the house because obviously that's where we're touching things the most and we don't know who has washed their hands or not. But in terms of like my room, it's kind of messy, because obviously, no one's going to come in the house and like, hang out with you. It's just you and like, whoever's living with you. No one's going to be barging in the room all the time. So, it's been kind of unkempt in here. But the rest of my house is really nice. [Laughter]

What do you think the city of Lowell or the federal government can or should do to keep residents safe and healthy during the pandemic?

What can they do to help keep the residents safe? I definitely think they should limit things that are open because even though they do want the economy to keep going, at the end of the day, you're still risking the health of these individuals. And I feel like that's a huge part in why our cases are still rising. Like Lowell right now is a red zone. They had to send all the kids back home, and it's difficult because there are kids who need to be in school. Right now, they only have the special needs kids in school because of course, they need to be there. But there's other kids who do need additional assistance who are sent home, and it is hard for parents who are working all the time to be there and help them out because they can't, they have to sustain a living for them.

It's crazy because I work in the Target at the CVS pharmacy. There are days where there's so many people in the store and it's congested. And that's not a great sign and because there's so many people, it's definitely going to be transmission of the virus quickly and rapidly. So, I think the city or like, the government should limit it again and then have stores limit how many people can go in because the stores say that they do limit people, but they don't. You know, there are days when they do but most of the time they don't. It's such a risk to do that. Because at the end of day, yes, you're getting money. But how much money can you make to lose a life of a person? You know, it's not worth it, in my opinion. So that's how I feel what the city should do.

So do you have any questions you'd like to ask me?

I guess for you because we live in two different cities—I'm from Lowell and you're from North Reading—how do you think the pandemic affected your surrounding areas, or affected you?

Well, I obviously live in a slightly different neighborhood than you do. Whereas yours is a little bit more urbanized, I live in the suburbs. So, for me, my closest neighbor is close by, but we all have huge yards where we can walk around, and I have trails behind my house that we walk through, and I live next to a pond I can walk around. I live on a dead-end street—basically, my neighborhood is a dead end, there's only one way in and one way out.

So, it affected me in a way that allowed me to maintain my lifestyle. I can still go for a run in the same place, I exercise in the same place, I do the same normal things as to where I walk my animals, where I go out. I think it was a bit different for me because I don't deal with as much congestion as someone from Lowell would, and the stores near my house—like for the first few months there were huge lines outside and that really quickly died down. Like you said, stores don't have people checking anymore, they had people at the door at first checking to make sure that they didn't hit the maximum amount of people all at once.

Also, it's a little different for me because I live in a mostly White town that is a higher tax bracket than most of the places. I definitely notice a lot of conservatives that don't want to wear masks. If they do wear masks, it's under their nose or on their chin, which doesn't do any good. [Laughter] It is interesting to see the differences because I feel like in cities the people are a bit more considerate, versus small towns, it's not as considerate which is odd to say or say or think. Is there anything we didn't discuss that you'd like to add?

I guess like the percentages of who has caught Covid in Lowell. So right now, of the majority of people in Lowell who have contracted Covid, I think half of them are Asian. And a majority of them are all minorities. So, it's Asians, Hispanics, and the Black community, a majority of that minority group has contracted Covid more than the White community. Obviously, Lowell has a large population of Cambodian, like Southeast Asian, individuals. And from my experience, and a majority of like, older, Cambodian generations, people that I know, I feel like a lot of people here don't have the ability to work from home. Because a lot of them don't speak English that well, so they can't get jobs where they can work from home and stay quarantined, which is unfortunate. You know, that goes for my parents. They can't stay home and work. My mom has a lot of body aches. My dad, he's been smoking for thirteen years. So, who knows, he's never been to the doctor for almost thirteen years, so I don't know if he's doing well with his health. And they always have to go in every day to work, of course with masks, but they're so susceptible to gaining the virus that it's unfortunate that they have to go through that.

The fact that a lot of people in these communities, not just in the Asian community, have to go in, it's sad to see that, you know, especially when they've been here for so long, and they have to go to work in such a global crisis right now. It's sad to see, you know, like, every day, you have to wonder, Are they okay? Are they going to get it? For myself, too. I have to watch out because I work at a pharmacy. I interact with sick people all the time. Of course, I take highly precautious measures, but at the end of the day, you never know what can happen.

Okay. Is there anything else you want to bring up?

I guess for you, do you know the percentages of who has con-tracted Covid in North Reading, like the different groups or the different areas where it, I guess like a hotspot, because you know, in Lowell there's Highlands and Pawtucketville, and such like that?

Well, like I said, North Reading is differently set up. It's all suburbs. So, there's not really official neighborhoods that we could kind of break that data up by, and honestly, I don't know who and how many people in North Reading have gotten Covid. I don't know. I think that also has to do with the income tax bracket, because most people don't have to go to work. I personally do have to work because I'm a server and a bartender.

But my parents, they work from home. My mother works for the Social Security Department and my father was a consultant for a major company until they hired him on and he's based out in California. So, it's a little bit different for me. I was able to be out of work for the three months implemented unemployment that we had, and I was comfortable being out of work because my parents were working still, and we all got to stay at home for three months. I was able to do that, and I was lucky to do that. I didn't feel lucky at first because I was bored out of my mind, but I was lucky enough to be able to do that. I think that there's definitely, right there, there's a class disparity. I definitely grew up privileged. And, you know, that's just how things worked out for my family. We were lucky and we got to stay home.

Obviously, my uncle, the one who was in Dracut, he had Covid. He's a veteran. He has all the predispositions that you can imagine. He had Covid for three weeks—he was in a coma for three weeks and intubated three weeks. So, it's like even though he's part of my family, it was a difference of even location, too, because he lived right outside of Lowell. And Lowell is a hotspot, and his roommate got it and then he got it. And it is what it is. They weren't able to stay home, or they didn't stay home. Or however they got it. I don't really know the full details or story.

So, I think that with my places, I have different privileges, just from where I grew up, who my family was, what my family does for work. I asked my parents if I should go back to work. It wasn't like, "I need to go back to work." It was "Should I go to work." Versus my parents were like, "Yeah, go ahead." There's no pressure on me to leave the house and go to work. So, I was afforded that, and I was lucky.

Wow. Yeah, I'd say there's definitely a huge difference in terms of me and you, because when the whole pandemic started, I had no choice to stop working, because obviously, I work in the pharmacy. Even with my parents, even though they knew what was going on, because we come from a low-middle class family, they're like, I don't care. If the pandemic is happening, you still need to work, which obviously didn't hurt me because they always said that to me. And I know that I need to kind of work to sustain myself, because I can't always rely on them to help me. I never was like that growing up.

But hearing that from them, it kind of hurt a little bit because it shows how not well-off we are as a family if they want me to continue to work and put myself out there with all these people coming in. Especially at the time, there was so many people coming in and asking, "Are you guys doing Covid testing?" when my location didn't do it. So, we had so many people

who could have had the virus just coming into the store filled with people asking if we can get a Covid test when we didn't do Covid tests there. That was already a huge indicator that what is happening right now is super dangerous.

So, I think that just thinking about that in the beginning was kind of emotional because you don't realize where you are, I guess, in the class structure until something like this happens. Because you don't have a choice. You have to do it. You can't just be like I'm going to stay home, which I feel goes for a majority of people in Lowell.

Is there anything else you want to discuss?

Hmmm. Oh my god. I did, I did have something to discuss and it left my brain. I guess like, for you, I have a question for you. What do you think of the government and the states still having things open or still wanting to have things open, especially when things are on the rise again? Or keeping things still at the same phase, what do you think of that?

They don't care that it's worse. That's exactly how I feel about these mandates is that they don't care that it is worse. The people that are passing these mandates and the people that are pushing for them especially, are privileged people, people who aren't going to be affected, they are demanding goods and services, and they get to go home. They get to choose to go out. Versus, say for example, I am a bartender and a server. I interact with, how many people in a week? How many people do I see a week, and do I serve in a week? And we got lucky, at my workplace we only had one Covid case. But the thing is, our work did not tell us, until two weeks after it happened.

Yeah, I definitely relate to that, because my sister's husband, in June, he doesn't work there anymore, but at the time he worked at an elderly residential housing. He was the maintenance manager there and they separated the patients—no, residents—the residents by floor. They separated the residents who had Covid onto one floor, and then those who did not onto separate floors. But, obviously going back to these companies not taking active precautions with what's going on. There was a resident, who was a Covid patient, who left their room and he somehow got to a floor that was non-Covid, saw my brother-in-law, and some of his coworkers, and sneezed on them. They contracted Covid. Of course, the company was at fault for that because they did not handle it correctly. They didn't isolate those residents as they should.

My brother-in-law was going to come home that night, told my sister, and my sister was like "No, you can't come home. Even though you got tested, you don't know what that result is yet." So, for about a month and a half, my nephews were almost fatherless that whole time. They couldn't see their dad. So, obviously, it affects—they're always asking, "Where's dad, where's dad?" Especially kids at that age, when you're so used to seeing your dad and having him be there for you, and have him gone, without him really saying bye to you.

It kind of hurts seeing them ask for him and only able to speak to him on the phone. And that stinks. Going back to the whole family thing, obviously it took a toll on my sister because raising three kids by yourself isn't fun. You know, with all of them in school and all of them being rambunctious little boys, it's not going to be a great time for her. So, I think that that was a big eventful thing that happened during the summer, during this pandemic, seeing that. I've always helped with my nephews, but, going back into that, because I've been a father figure to them too, it feels weird. Yeah.

Anything else you want to say?

I think that's it.

Okay, thank you for participating in this. I really appreciated this conversation. Thank you so much.

***

Update

I graduated from UMass Lowell in December, 2021, with a degree in biology. Currently, I'm the director for my dance team, INC, based in Boston and pursuing my endeavors on going to medical school—William Chan

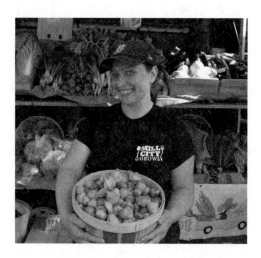

Jessica Wilson

"I mean, the people of America are our people, their health is our health. If people need food, they should be given food. If people need a place to live, they should be given a place to live. If people need help with their children, they should be given help with their children, and those are things that the government can provide when the market can't—I think that's the responsibility."

Jessica Wilson is a forty-two-year-old woman of French-Canadian descent who is the current executive director of Mill City Grows, a nonprofit food justice organization in Lowell. She was born in Lowell and grew up in both Lowell and Dracut, leaving the area to go to college and graduate school, and then returning to Lowell in 2006 to work at local non-profits. She lives in Tyngsboro with her husband, Peter, and daughter, River. In her interview, Jessica discusses challenges and creative responses to both managing Mill City Grows and life at home during the pandemic, as well as broader food justice and social equity issues.

Jessica Wilson was interviewed by Jenna Solomine on November 20, 2020.

Okay, now we'll talk about your experiences during the pandemic. So how has your life changed during the current Covid-19 pandemic?

In every way imaginable. I actually just started this job in January, as the executive director of Mill City Grows. I've worked with the organization for four years. It was co-founded by two wonderful and great friends of mine. One of them is a UMass alum, Lydia Sisson. The other one is Francey Slater. Both of them had experience in the food world and they asked me to come be a part of Mill City Grows as a volunteer when they started it ten years ago, which I did. And then I joined the staff to help out with some development work about four years ago when I was pregnant with my daughter. And you know, as she got older, I started working more and more and I loved the work. I love the organization and they both had stated a few years ago to me that they were interested in moving on and not working day-to-day in the organization for personal reasons. I had experience as a nonprofit executive director in the past. So I thought it would be a great opportunity for me to use that skill set and get back into the full-time workforce and lead this organization that I love so much.

So, January started out normal, like, okay, taking on a new job, new leadership position, and pretty quickly in March, we realized something wasn't quite right. And within the first two weeks of March everything about the operations of this organization, which I've been involved with for ten years, had to change rapidly and completely. We were going with the Centers for Disease Control and Prevention (CDC) guidance at the time, the information that was coming out from the state, which was changing every day. I will say, it was a three-week period where literally, I feel like I spent every day from the moment I woke up to the moment I went to bed, trying to process the new information I was getting about this pandemic, figure out what that meant for the safety and well-being of my team, and then how to translate that into a policy. I remember every week on Friday, for a month or so just literally feeling like my body would like (gestures downward with hand) plunk. You know, I just had nothing left. And I was like, okay, I need two days to not think about work, hopefully, nothing terrible happens in the world, and I'll get back to it on Monday. So, I think that stepping into a job where I thought I knew what I was doing, I had experience, and I felt really confident and excited, and then to have all of that just erased in a couple of days. And like, okay, we're in a brand-new playing field, the game is brand new. You're not sure what the rules are. Good luck. That's kind of how it felt for a while.

At home my husband and I both work full time. I do this job. He's an engineer. And our daughter was in full-time daycare. So, she had a forty-hour week job too. We dropped her off and picked her up, and her daycare closed. And so, she's been at home with us as we do these jobs ever since. Both my husband and I, our jobs are considered essential. So, we do go into the office. And we take turns obviously, we're not both in the office at the same time. One of us always has to be at home with our child. So that means that, you know, some workdays are, there's a lot of playing on the floor with blocks. And other days, I have meetings, and I can't cancel them, I have a little helper back here, flicking the lights on and off or over at that table doing crafts. But the mornings tend to be better than the afternoon. So she's pretty occupied right now. After lunchtime I try not to schedule any meetings because, I'm serious, like all hell breaks loose. And it's like Romper Room in here. She's only one child, but she feels like ten, all over the place. I think in the personal and professional, it's been pretty amazingly different. And I think like eight months in now, we've created a lot of new ways of doing things. I mean, none of it feels normal. But it all feels a lot more do-able today than it did eight months ago, you know, for better or worse.

Yeah, hopefully this new normal doesn't have to go on for too much longer.

It doesn't have to be normal. I think it's the new what we're doing. I refuse to call it the new normal because none of this is normal. And none of it is okay.

How would you describe what a typical day is like for you now compared to before the pandemic?

So, I wouldn't say my life before the pandemic was super easy, right? We were a very busy family, and the place where I work is a very busy workplace. We run a lot of different programs. And so, we very much operate on the cycle of the seasons, too. We're ramping things up in the spring, we're growing and harvesting and distributing all summer and fall, and then at this time of year, late November, we start wrapping things up, closing up our outdoor spaces, preparing for the winter and planning for next year. So, I mean, that hasn't changed, I think the pace of our work has remained the same.

What did change is the way that our workdays are like—we were very much a team that works together, we're out working the land together. My function is not to be a full-time farmer. But I do participate in that work. And so, I think the thing that's been really hard is that we have some of our team that are central and do have to go in every day, and some of our team that we're telling them, they have to stay home. That disconnect makes things very hard. As a person who works in nonprofits who kind of understands culture is the success of an organization, we've worked really hard to build a very strong culture at Mill City Grows, where we all really understand what each other does, we all participate in each other's jobs. So, I'm not a farmer, but I farm with my team. The people who don't work in the gardens, they're not gardeners and community advocates and community organizers. But we do that work and support it, too. It's been really challenging to find ways for us to overlap and intersect in this environment where we can't be together, we can't touch each other, we can't share food and cook for one another, as much as we want to. And we can't see the people who participate in our programs. You know, we're so far away from that. We usually do a lot of classes, we have activities, we'll have groups of dozens of volunteers come to our farm. So we've been able to do a little bit of that safely through the year when numbers were lower, and restrictions were a little bit looser, we were able to do some group work with social distance. But I think that lack of interaction has been the biggest difference and trying to find substitutes for that.

We had a practice at one point where we took turns, a member of our team every day would send out an email to everyone on the team, kind of like an inspirational email and it could be whatever you wanted. It could be a picture of your kids, a poem, a video, a song, an idea. We did that for a few months. And it was actually a really nice way to keep in touch with each other, keep the morale up and just remind ourselves why we're here. We used to meet as a staff once a month. We started doing that once a week on Zoom, because we didn't see each other, so we wanted to all see each other's faces at least once a week. So that's been really important and just kind of updating each other. We've celebrated birthdays on Zoom; we have this really weird tradition where we all sing happy birthday on Zoom. And because of delays it's absolutely terrible. But we love doing it. So, we do that a lot. We did get together once, as a staff at the farm during the summer. That was the only time we've all been at the same space all year long, and it was really nice. We had our masks on, and we each brought our own food and just had a little kind of harvest celebration. So those are the things that have been really different.

In my personal life, and I think every family has done a version of this, my husband and I had to have a really serious discussion about what this was going to mean for our family. Whether or not we wanted to try to find daycare for our child once daycare opened back up, and we decided not to. We had to think about how we were going to see our family, if we were going to see our family, what safety meant, and how we were going to divide certain tasks in a different way than we had before. Those were all really hard discussions to have, because we're in this environment of heightened stress and kind of uncertainty, but being able to have the conversations has been the thing that's really gotten us successfully to this point where we're both still employed, we're both still speaking to each other. And with love, and I think that I really believe very strongly in the concept that you can have post-traumatic stress and you can have post-traumatic growth, and everybody has within them the ability to turn trauma into growth, but you really do have to have the resources available to you. You have to be surrounded by people who care about you, and you have to care about them. You have to have the resources of being able to communicate your needs clearly. And you have to also really believe that there's something better on the other side.

As tough as it has been, and we have been through some, like, we've had some really bad days in my house, we both feel strongly that we're committed to this relationship and this family. And so, we've taken this opportunity to grow as a couple, and really listen to each other better and care about each other. I wish we didn't have to go through this to get there. But I see that as a gift that my husband and I have given to each other. We never took our stress out on each other. We always really talked about it, and I don't think I would have been able to do this job and be a leader, if I didn't have a partner who cared about me so much. I probably would have quit my job. You know I think I would have had to, because I think it's just, a human being can only deal with so much. I think it's certainly been very different in both personal life and work. But I think some good things have come.

That's actually kind of a part of the next question. Are there any positive aspects to your life during the pandemic?

Well, I think what I just shared, having to be creative about communication, and then coming up with these great ways to keep in touch with people you don't see or creating new ways of communicating with the people you see, like, way more than you were anticipating. But I think the one thing, and this is something that I actually have to remind myself of every day, my daughter is very little, and she's growing and changing so much every day. She'll be four in January. And if she was in full-time daycare, and I was working full-time, and things were normal, and I was going out to events two or three nights a week, because that's what you do when you work in nonprofit in Lowell—I wouldn't have been able to be with her so much. I have spent so much time with her this year. So much more than I have since she was an infant, and I was on maternity leave. In the past few years, the only times I've spent that much time with her is when we take a family vacation. And I will say it's a lot to get used to, to be with the toddler, alone all day. But I've gotten to know her at this really incredible time in her life, that as a working mom, I never would have had that opportunity.

And I see how in many ways I'm very lucky. I have a job where I'm in charge, I have ultimate flexibility for my schedule. I have been able to create a work environment where other parents are dealing with these challenges. I've given them the flexibility to stay home if they need to and shift their work hours. And I've been able to have afternoons where I said, Okay, it's three o'clock, I'm gonna take a couple hours off of work, because I know I'm coming back to it at 8 p.m. And I'm going to go take my kid on a hike, and we're going to just spend some time together. We've done a lot of that this year. And I've honestly cherished every moment I've had with her even in the moments where

I'm like losing my mind because she's asking me why for the fifty-seventh time in the row, or she won't eat the meal that I've prepared for her or we're hiking in the woods, and she tells me she needs to go the bathroom and we're like twenty minutes away from a bathroom and I didn't bring any towels. You know, there's all that. And there's just the constant existential crisis of like, oh my god, the world is ending. But I would never have had that time with her. And she will never be this age again. And I have had the great honor and privilege to be able to educate and raise my three-year-old to a four-year-old as a working mom running a business. Like who gets to do that? I mean, I know why people don't do it because it's hard and awful, but I got to do it. And I think that's probably for me, the best thing that I can say has happened this year.

That's a really good thing it sounds like. So, if you ever needed help, maybe with your daughter or work, how did you receive help when you needed it?

A lot of the help I needed, I think, was just somebody to talk to. And I, again, I'm very lucky and very privileged and very thankful that we have great relationships with all of our family. So, my personal family, my in-laws, I've always been able to pick up the phone and call them. There have been occasions where I do need childcare. But nobody is available to come to my house. So, I've been able to call up my sister in-law and put her on a FaceTime call with my daughter for thirty minutes while I go do something, which those things have been great. We have had grandparent visits in the yard. And I literally have had grandparents come over and be like, okay, you're going to play ball in the yard for an hour, I'm going to go do a meeting and I'll be back.

And I think we've had our own medical scares, we've had a Covid exposure—we haven't had it ourselves, but we had some medical issues. So, I work for a company that gives health care, I have access to a doctor, I have transportation, and I have money to pay my copay. So, like, those things were accessible to me. And I do the job that I do, because I know that that's not the situation for everyone. I think the one time this year where I wasn't able to get what I needed was right at the beginning, when everybody was afraid to go to the store. When you went to the store, there wasn't necessarily always food there. There were literally a couple weeks where I just kind of let the food run out because I didn't know what to do. And it wasn't a question of whether or not we could afford it because we were both employed adults. It was just like, I don't have time to go to the store. I don't want to go to the store, I'm afraid, I can't get anybody to deliver food to my house, because there's no availability of that service. What am I going to do? And one of my coworkers actually brought me a box of food. And this is kind of ironic as someone who runs farms, I hadn't had a fresh vegetable in a week. And it was like there was lettuce in there and potatoes and some citrus fruit. And I was just like, Oh my god, this is the best thing that's ever happened to me. I couldn't explain to you how thankful I was and how excited I was to eat romaine lettuce, I was just so excited. And I remember making a salad for me and my husband was like, "Isn't this good? Isn't this amazing? Don't you feel so healthy." And that, you know, as things have changed and improved, and we kind of know more things now than we did then, I've been keeping us fed.

But I feel like it gave me this moment where it reminded me why I work at Mill City Grows, and why we do this work. I experienced this once. There are people whose entire lives are about trying to find the resources they need to keep their family healthy. And there are not enough ways to provide those things for them in this country, this rich, wonderful, beautiful country that we have. And I have continued doing my job this year. I have been so inspired by my team, because that is the gap we are filling, right, we are giving the help to people that need it, we are making sure that at this time when our personal health is so important, and one of the factors of personal health is that you're able to eat a healthy, nutritious diet. We're allowing that to be possible for hundreds and hundreds and hundreds of people. I think I cherished that help that I received at this moment when I needed it when I wasn't asking for it, you know, because I didn't know how, I never had before. I've never had to ask anybody for help getting food before, that's never been a part of my life. And so to be given it so freely by somebody who cared about me, and to know that that's what I was doing for other people, I think has been a really an important lesson for me and just an important feeling to know that my work has value for people and that there may be somebody out there that feels as good as I felt when I received that box. You know, it's pretty cool.

What are your thoughts about mask wearing?

I love it. We have been wearing masks since it was possible to sew a mask. I think it was like anything we could do to protect ourselves and our child and anybody we were seeing I was totally for. We have a giant box of masks in our entryway. So, we always grab them before we go out. I have a little pouch with my spare masks in it in my pocketbook, just so I'm never without one. And I know that it's not 100 percent effective. And I know that wearing it doesn't mean that you won't get sick. But to me, it feels like there's one more thing I can do to protect myself and others. And I will do that. We actually have this really cool collection of masks like we have masks that people have made for us. We have masks that we bought from local businesses. We have masks that we've purchased as part of fundraising campaigns. My daughter really likes Paw Patrol. So, I got her a set of Paw Patrol masks. And even though she's really little, and according to our current advisory, she's not required to wear one because she's not five yet, we go to the playground sometimes. I always say if you're going to see other kids, we never know what's going to happen, you should keep your mask on. I think seeing us do it, she's really good at it. And so that kind of makes me happy because it is unpleasant. I mean, it's unpleasant to have a thing on your face, especially if you're trying to run around and play or do anything physical. And you have this barrier to breathing. Like it's not fun. But I think the message that I give to her, and that I tell myself is that this is one more thing we can do to stay healthy and help other people stay healthy. And hopefully this will be done at some point in the near future, if we do these things.

You received a Covid test, how did that go?

We got two because we were exposed to a neighbor who had a positive test. We found out the next day, and, it was a low-risk kind of thing, but we were just kind of freaked out. So, I had two successive tests, one immediately and then I waited another five days. Another one I went to a drive- thru testing site at Circle Health and made an appointment. As I told you, I have health insurance. I wasn't worried about not being able to pay for it. And it hurt. But it was fine. And I got my results pretty rapidly because this happened over the summer so there weren't four hour waits to get tests and things. But I guess every nurse does this differently, the first one wasn't so bad. The second one was incredibly painful. And I remember I pulled my mask down, they stick this thing up your nose. And I was just like, oh, and the nurse was pretty funny, she was like, "Just make sure you're done crying before you drive away." Like that was unnecessary. But it was kind of funny. So yeah, I never had any symptoms, of course, and I tested negative both times, but it's just a weird thing. You drive up to this parking spot, you open your door, this masked stranger that's dressed in a spacesuit comes and sticks a pipe cleaner up your nose. And then you drive away.

Have things been different for you in terms of self-care and cleaning your house?

That is a funny question. Well, not really. I don't get dressed up very often, but I have a couple of times, less than a couple times a week. But every once in a while, I'm like, I'm going to put makeup on, just because I feel like it. We've done a few virtual events at work. So, we actually constructed this beautiful kitchen at Mill City Grows, which we wanted to do community education and we haven't done that yet. And we wanted to do a grand opening, because lots of people gave us money to build this kitchen. So we did a grand opening on Zoom, and I actually got dressed up and put makeup on and wore red lipstick. And I was like, I haven't done this in months, it's so much fun.

Even though I haven't left the house, I've still had a few occasions. So that's actually been really nice. I have gotten my hair cut a few times this year, which was a fun experience. And I think I really reflected a lot on my experiences as a new mother when I was on maternity leave. As someone who has been a career woman, until I gave birth to my daughter at thirty-nine or thirty-eight, I can't remember how old I was. But that was a huge shift for me. One of the pieces of advice I had received from a nurse was, don't be uncomfortable, but get dressed and have a shower, feed yourself. Because these are the things that are going to make you feel good and make you feel normal, as you're getting used to this new way of living. I feel like that advice has really rung in my head through this process. Like, this is a new way of living. You have to remember that you still need to feel good, you still need to be able to function, you still need to be healthy to do the things you need to do. So yes, I put clothes on every day, I get showered every day.

As for cleaning the house, I think for months, I was obsessively cleaning the house. And we have a child. I think that one of the things we've kind of compromised on is, you need to pick your battles when you have a toddler, where before I think we were very specific, like, every night before you go to bed, we have to clean up all the toys. You know, there have been nights where I don't want to fight with anybody about this. And honestly, I don't care, just kick the toys over to the side of the room. We'll deal with it tomorrow. So certainly, knowing that nobody is coming over, the level of clutter we allow is whatever. But we have still decorated for holidays and done things like that. One of the things I actually really enjoy doing with my daughter-- she likes doing the things that I do, so she has a little mop and she cleans the kitchen floor. So, we try to integrate that into our daily routine, even if it's not as thorough as it once was. But yeah, I think that we certainly wear more sweatpants than we did before.

What do you think the city of Lowell and/or the federal government can and should do to help keep residents safe and healthy?

I think you will see where my heart and politics are with this answer. I think that we need consistent messaging on what we're supposed to do. While I understand this is a free country, I feel in an emergency situation, we need rules and regulations, and we should be asked to follow them. So that is something the government should be doing for us and making those statements very clear. I also think that, and I think this anytime, people should be given the help they need to survive and also to live a healthy life. In instances where the market doesn't provide for that the government needs to. There shouldn't be any debate about this. These are our siblings, our family, the people that we care about. I mean, the people of America are our people, their health is our health. If people need food, they should be given food. If people need a place to live, they should be given a place to live. If people need help with their children, they should be given help with their children, and those are things that the government can provide when the market can't—I think that's the responsibility. I do my part, because I believe in this so strongly, and I swear to you, I have given a donation to every organization that's doing good work in this area, because I know how hard they're working, and how much their work is needed. It's just needed, like more than ever.

Thank you so much for doing this. Zoom hasn't cut us off yet.

Yeah, it could happen anytime—we usually get a little count-down when it starts to go. I had heard that, and I know it's not Thanksgiving weekend, but I had heard that Zoom was turning that off for Thanksgiving time so that families could connect more.

Do you have any questions you'd like to ask me or anything else that we didn't discuss that you would like to add?

I think this is a really awesome project. One of the ways we do our evaluation at Mill City Grows is through storytelling, because I think it captures better what the impact of the work we do actually is. I think data is really important. And statistics are really important because they kind of show at this macro level, but it's really these personal stories where you understand the full impact of what you do. It's so important to be able to let people tell you their stories in their own words. I think it's a pretty cool thing.

Specifically in Lowell, you're going to get much richer stories if you can have multiple language capacity. Because, I'm sure you may have heard this, we have over forty percent, I think, of people that live in Lowell, who were born in a country other than the United States. And so maybe twenty or twenty-five percent of high school students are English language learners, so I feel with older folks, that percentage will be even higher. I know we have a couple of staff who are bilingual, and one of the women I work with always says, "Sometimes I need to write down what I want to say in Spanish. And then I tell it to you in English, my brain just works better that way." So, I think if you have the capacity, and you can give this feedback to folks,

I think being able to do that would be incredible. And you'll definitely have a much richer archive with that. I say this as a person with a long history of working deeply in communities in Lowell. I am clearly a White person, I speak English, English is my native language, so these are all things I have learned by working in the community and with other people, too.

Well, it was so nice talking to you, Jenna. This was really fun.

This was a great interview, thank you so much!

***

Update

I am still working as the Executive Director at Mill City Grows, and still working with the community to ensure food access for those who continue to need assistance. My husband and I are working in our respective offices much more now, though working from home remains an at least weekly activity for both of us. My daughter started preschool in September 2021. She loves it, and her teachers and schoolmates mean the world to her. We've had three Covid quarantines since school began, but luckily no Covid, and since River turned five in January, now my entire family is vaccinated! We're slowly, safely, making get-togethers with friends and family part of our routine again, but it still feels so different. We've all been through something major, and that is going to take a long time to fully process—Jessica Wilson

5.

Community Organizations and Mutual Aid

Carina Pappalardo
Psychological Center Chief Executive Officer, Lawrence

Vilma Martínez-Dominguez
Community Development Director, City of Lawrence

Felicia Sullivan
non-profit researcher, member of Lifting Lowellians: Assistance and Mutual Aid (LLAMA), Lowell

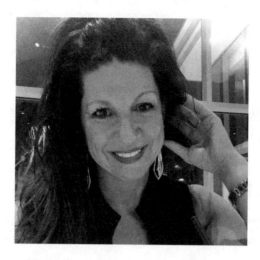

Carina Pappalardo

"How can you give up on somebody's life? You can't."

Carina Pappalardo is the Chief Executive Officer for The Psychological Center in Lawrence, Mass., which offers two residential recovery programs for women (Pegasus House and Women's View) and a shelter for men and women experiencing homelessness (Daybreak Shelter). She is forty-seven years old and describes herself as American of Italian and French heritage.

Carina was interviewed by Phillips Academy students Emilia S. and Bryan J. on May 6, 2020.

Hi, my name is Carina Pappalardo. I am The Psychological Center's Chief Executive Officer. I was born June 24, 1973, here in Methuen, Mass., actually that's where my hometown is. I've always been a girl from the Merrimack Valley. My profession prior to this has always been business-related and in human resources. I do have my bachelor's degree from the University of Massachusetts Lowell, and my master's degree from Western New England College.

You said that you were from Methuen. How did you get involved with Lawrence?

So as a city, you know, growing up in the Merrimack Valley I've visited Lawrence many times. My grandmother lived in Lawrence for an extremely long time, most of her life on Auburn Street prior to moving to Methuen herself. The connection was just always staying local to the Merrimack Valley, which was something that I was always interested in when finding employment as well. You know, I wasn't interested in commuting to Boston and spending hours on the road, it was more of being local, helping people in the Merrimack Valley, and still being able to maintain a close distance to family.

How did you become involved with The Psychological Center?

So back in 2010, I was working at a prior company and they were doing some restructuring, and part of that was having to relocate, which I wasn't interested in. So you know, thinking that it was the end of the world and what was I going to do, what was going to be next for me in my life, I applied on Indeed.com for a position here at The Psychological Center in the Human Resources department. My first ever nonprofit that I worked for, but I was like, How different can it be, you know? It's nonprofit, but how different can it be? And sure enough it was actually quite different compared to working for for-profit businesses. So still being interested in staying local, I was really excited to come on, not just for something different, but to work with individuals in the population that I have never worked with before, being on the addiction piece and the homelessness piece. So I was really excited about that opportunity.

You wanted me to talk a little bit about the programs themselves. You know people will often say to me, "How do you do it?" And you know there's a lot of negativity that people see in the news when it comes to addiction or to mental health or to homelessness, and quite honestly I really truly feel that I'm one of the luckiest people, because I'm blessed to be able to work with individuals who inspire me, inspire my staff, they bring such great hope to a population that could easily give up. And they fight every single day. So when we talk about the programs that we have, Pegasus House and Women's View, first, they're pretty similar; they're both female residential recovery programs. These are for ladies who are struggling with an addiction to drugs, alcohol, or a combination. All have mental health issues as well, and that is usually associated to prior severe traumatic events that have happened in their lives, typically at a very early age you know, we're talking about five, six, seven years old maybe earlier, for the most part. And these might have been attributed to physical violence, emotional abuse, sexual abuse. They all have their different stories but many of them have a lot of similarities.

So there's fifteen beds in each program. The biggest difference between the two programs is that Pegasus House is for females eighteen to twenty-five years old. Women's View is for females over the age of twenty-five. Structurally though they're both set up the same. There's a lot of work. I always say we're not a five-star hotel. We're not concierge services. They work very hard from the minute they get up until when they go to bed. There's individual counseling, there's group counseling, life skill building throughout the day. Chores that they have to do. We don't cook for them. We don't clean for them. We don't do their laundry. In addition to working on their mental health and their addiction, it's that life skills piece. A lot of it too is teaching them how to go to the grocery store or how to budget their bank accounts. You know things that they may have never been taught while they were growing up.

What has your experience been with the current crisis and what's going on and how has the atmosphere changed? What is the mood around these programs and The Psychological Center?

Yes, and I'll get to Daybreak Shelter as well, but to answer that question it's been really difficult for them because they look forward to going on pass. And typically during the pass they get to see their families. They get to see their children. And we haven't been able to allow them to do that because of the social distancing and the quarantines. Going to meetings actually has been different for them too, and that's a big part of their recovery. They were going to meetings every single day—they can't, we're doing those through Zoom so that they're not in that large gathering, so that's changed for them, too. Health and wellness is a really big part of these programs. They go to the gym every day. They haven't been able to go to the gym so that's changed for them. We're trying to just do some fitness that we can at the program, obviously on a much smaller scale. So, for us we find that it may be challenging and difficult to go through this quarantine or social distance, right, and isolate ourselves from people, but for them the magnitude is much greater because they're already working on something so hard, and change is really, really difficult or can be really difficult to them. So that entire lifestyle change is affecting them at this point.

As for Daybreak Shelter, it is a homeless shelter here in Lawrence and we have fifty beds. Typically it's thirty-five males, fifteen females. We're in a very small area. There's no place inside that building to isolate anybody from somebody else, so I think that through some leadership decisions and some teamwork, the collaboration and partners within the city, we've been able to, for the most part, keep any positive cases at bay and we did so for quite a bit of time. We did have a few cases and then those people we were able to find isolation centers through the state in Lexington, Mass. And right now what we've done is put up some shower curtains between the bunk beds. The bunk beds are really close together—where someone sleeps, if you reach your hand out you can pretty much feel the person sleeping next to you, that's how close the bunk beds are. So it's been quite challenging there, but we have been very diligent in all of the sanitizing and making sure that we have all of the protective equipment—the gloves, the masks, and cleaning constantly. The guests there for the most part have been remarkable. They understand what we're doing. There really hasn't been any pushback to it. They stay with us during the day now. Typically, our guests would leave at 8 a.m. and come back at 4 p.m. so we're running that around the clock, they're not leaving they're staying, and they're really making the best of it. So my staff all around have been working really hard with trying to find some new fun ideas just to keep everybody occupied during the day.

What are some of those fun ideas that you do throughout the day?

They've been doing a lot of arts and crafts, and they've been trying to get outside, exercising, playing games, horseshoes, volleyball, basketball. Trying to find some of those typical yard games.

You mentioned that there's a thirty-five male to fifteen female ratio, why is that?

It's the way that the shelter itself is set up. They're actually modular trailers that you would see on the side of the road if there was some type of construction. When they put this in place they were building the new high school, and the administration at the time, the city council, and the high school administration decided that they would put these four trailers together. There's about 2,744 square feet, which is the size of a typical household for a family of four or family of five, so we have over fifty people plus staff in there. And the way that the trailers were set up at the time, and the way that the dorms are, there's one male dorm and it's much larger than the one female dorm, so that's how it split out. And then we actually put some mats on the floor sometimes if we need to take additional people in. You know safety first too, making sure that we're not blocking any exits or anything, but especially in the colder weather we want to make sure that we can get as many people in as possible. And with the females, I mean it happens to males as well, but with the females who might be escaping domestic violence situations, being prostituted, being trafficked, we want to make sure that we can get them inside safely.

What are some of the biggest challenges with this pandemic?

Space was the biggest challenge and immediately we tried to get a tent to put on our site at Daybreak Shelter, which was shot down by the city. The mayor didn't allow us to do that, he thought that it was going to be more dangerous and spreading the virus, which I have to respectfully disagree with. You know when we tried to consider the social distancing, I was never adding to the number that we had, I was only trying to separate them out, so space was a huge issue for us. And as I mentioned earlier it could have run rampant in the very beginning and gone through the entire fifty guests that we had plus the staff members, and if they all became positive and we didn't have any place to isolate them then that's just more people that would have been out there on the streets spreading the virus. So space was definitely the biggest challenge that we faced. Luckily, we were able to hang in there and utilize some other resources, so at this point, we feel we have overcome that challenge with the space. At least for this round. You know there's a lot of talk that this might subside, the virus may subside, and then come back in the fall. So, we're trying to figure out a solution should that happen again and be proactive with it if possible.

And in terms of the guests, are the majority of them from the Lawrence area or are they from other places?

Most of our guests I'd say are from the Lawrence area. Definitely throughout the Merrimack Valley as well we do see some guests. You know when we talk about the homeless shelter, at least when we talk about Daybreak Shelter, we are a state-funded program. We don't look at any type of geographic barrier, so if anyone comes to Lawrence for whatever reason, if they need us, then we're going to provide safe services for them.

What has your personal experience been with social distancing?

So we obviously are an essential business. We couldn't stop the programs, we weren't going to shut down. Now I sit in an administrative office, I could stay home and work out of my house, but because the administrative office is pretty isolated in and of itself, I have been coming in. I don't go to the programs. All of the meetings that I might have with the staff or checking in with the guests I do the same way as we are, virtually, just to make sure that everyone has everything that they need. Yeah and making sure that I wear that mask every time I go out if necessary. You know it's hard even for me as a person. I'm missing a lot of stuff that I would usually have in my life outside of work, and just trying to make the best of it as we get through this.

Of course, and is there anything you or maybe the guests didn't expect they would miss?

The biggest thing that they ask me is, "When can we go out Carina? We want to go out." So they miss that. When they're used to a specific structure and a specific routine, and then that changes, it's difficult. And we try to not change it overnight— we held off as long as we could, still based with the governor's recommendations, we really held off not letting them go out for quite some time. But that's been the biggest challenge. The biggest obstacle for them is not being able to see their family. We try to connect them through Zoom, but it's not, you know, with that population it's not as easy to do as it is for us to just connect with Zoom. We didn't have a lot of the technology in place, you know, whether it was laptops or computers, so we are trying to bring in some more Smart TVs and webcams and laptops. Because we can't stop—you know the coronavirus is not going to stop us from the programming that we have. So really just putting those pieces in place was really important, but that was definitely the biggest obstacle.

How do you keep pushing forward and instill this kind of mood for your guests?

At the end of the day, it's always about the guests. So, you know nothing's gonna get me down whether it's a big rainstorm or snowstorm or something that tries to interfere with how we operate. You know, there was one video that I put out earlier a few weeks ago saying that we're still weathering the storm without this tent because at the end of the day these people need us. There's absolutely no way I would ever give up in trying to provide or giving them what they deserve and part of that is just dignity and respect, and we will do whatever it takes to make sure that that continues. Just because they're struggling in life right now—it can be any of us—you know people often will say, "Oh you know, what's the type of person that you usually see there?" And I said "It could be anyone. It could be anyone in my family, your family. Look around when you're at the mall it could be anybody that you see in public." There are no barriers to who might be affected from the mental health or addiction or homelessness, so I just always have operated that way—that people matter. And I would never give up on trying to protect the people that are so vulnerable regardless if I'm told no a hundred times, I'm still going to protect them.

What do you think is going to be a challenge when this crisis ends?

You know, I feel really bad for the individuals who might be housed right now who were on the street. So, I'm not talking about Daybreak Shelter, because anybody from Daybreak Shelter may have gone to one of the isolation centers that the state put on like in Lexington. We do have a few individuals over at the hotel in Andover that the city contracted with, they will all come back to us. It's the individuals that were outside that are now inside, you know what is the plan going to be for them? You know, where are they going to go? So, I just hope that there's a lot of thought put in for those particular individuals and hopefully they can get some more services to them, that's important.

Would you say there's a lot of cooperation from neighboring cities and towns?

For us and for the people who are outside in the city of Lawrence, because that's all I really know, I'm not sure how it has been for—I mean I hear about Boston and Lowell—and it seems like they have a lot of opportunity. I feel like Lawrence was a little bit behind the eight ball when it came to this and getting these contracts in place with the two hotels. Andover I think went a little bit smoother than the one in Methuen went and they're accepting different populations and there was a lot of restrictions put into the hotels—who they would take and who they wouldn't take, so that was definitely one of biggest challenges. I think that it's fantastic though that the city of Methuen and that Andover was able to help in this situation.

Who will provide those services to people currently inside and otherwise outside?

That's a great question and it's probably one of the questions that we've been trying to figure out for a really long time. The homelessness issue and where can they go and who can help them and the space issues. Rents in the area are extremely high, I think that keeps a lot of people from being housed unfortunately. You know, whether landlords want to accept people who are coming from the street that might have not so good histories is a barrier for them as well. So I'm not positive. I just know that for the individuals who have been at Daybreak, we'll continue to provide those services. One of our goals is to get a much larger building so that we can assist more individuals. We just don't have the capacity. As a matter of fact, the state only funds us for thirty-eight of our beds so those other twelve beds that we fill are unfunded. We eat that cost by ourselves, that's why it's important for us to do fundraising and grant writing. We were supposed to have an event this past Saturday, May 2nd, it was going to be our fourth annual Kentucky Derby event and you know without being able to have that we don't have those additional funds coming in that we would typically have to help supplement the loss of the beds over at Daybreak Shelter. I would never, having the space, say, You know what, because you're only funding me for thirty-eight, I'm only gonna fill thirty-eight. That just would never sit right with me, so we continue to operate at full or over capacity so hopefully we can try to find a building that will allow us to help more individuals who are outside

Is there anything that you're doing now, that you hope to carry out with you back into normalcy once things go back to what they were once this crisis ends?

I think that the biggest shift in what we've had to do is the virtual. And it proves that we can probably have components of the virtual capacity in the programs for individuals who can continue telehealth services. So if we can't get someone in quickly to see a clinician or to see a medication prescriber, is there someone who might be further away from us distance-wise that our guests can just have a telehealth appointment with them? Because if we can open it up that way then that would be very useful to us as well as having 24/7 access to any type of recovery meeting. So not only just going out and having those meetings, but if someone is really struggling and can't get a hold of their sponsor then they can, you know, hopefully connect with someone via a virtual gateway and have the opportunity at that point. I think that's something that we can carry back into normalcy. Our programs are really focused on empowering people, so however we can continue empowering them. This was a blessing in disguise that we are now able to find new opportunities to continue that empowerment and build back that self-confidence in someone. And knowing that there are alternatives—when life throws you a curveball like this we don't sit back, we don't roll over, that we're going to figure it out. We're gonna forge ahead and come out better on the other side. The situation obviously is not ideal, but blessings in disguise with what we can do going forward.

What inspired you to tell your story to the Lawrence History Center? What inspired you to tell this to the public and for it to be recorded?

I think that it is a great opportunity for the public and every generation that will come afterwards to see how we were able to band together and pull through this and continue. Regardless of what's thrown our way, there's always a way to get ahead of something. Obstacles are going to always come in our life, this is just another obstacle. We suffered back in 2015 when we closed the Counseling Center, and it was pretty significant at that time, but we forged forward. The kind of programs that we have continue to thrive and we hope to move forward with new programs in the future. So telling the story is important so that it's just another reminder to people not to ever give up and by not giving up we are saving so many lives. And I think at the end of the day you know how can you give up on somebody's life? You can't. I think that's the biggest piece.

Thank you. Is there anything that you think we missed? Is there anything that you want to say too that we might not have covered right now?

I just want to say, when you asked me about why I wanted to

share this with the Lawrence History Center, it's important to let the community know what's going on. But I think that it's individuals like yourself and your peers over at Phillips. You're the next leaders, you know you are the ones who are gonna take over the world and you can shape how it continues to be. That is really important for me and I think that's another reason why I liked sharing this story so that you can see the human aspect of what's happening during this time. I appreciate what you and your peers will continue to provide in this world for all of these individuals who need help.

***

Update

It has been a few long years, with many days of exhaustion, but I am keeping up with positive energy. I am still as busy as ever with the three programs however, they all help lift me up, too. In any spare time I am fitting in exercising for my mental health or listening to music in my car. I am blessed for sure. Our agency has continued to fully operate throughout the start of the pandemic, the variants, and the unknowns to come. We have followed all of the recommendations and guidelines set forth by the Department of Public Health. We have offered vaccinations, booster shots, and Covid-19 related information to all of our guests. The biggest challenges we continue to face are exhaustion and a shortage of staff. However, our priority is safety for our current staff and guests. We continue to test all of our guests at least once a week and sometimes twice a week. This will go on for as long as necessary—Carina Pappalardo

Dear Charlotte,
May we always
take time to
listen and
learn from
sharing
stories.

Vilma Martinez-Dominguez

Vilma Martínez-Dominguez

"I don't think this is just a responsibility of our mayor or our administration but this is a civic responsibility. And I think that that's what made Lawrence the city that it is. Because we have a lot of partnerships, a lot of caring people. We have a lot of support, we have a lot of love for this city."

Vilma Martínez-Dominguez is the Community Development Director for the City of Lawrence and has spent her career empowering the citizens of Lawrence. She worked in various roles for the YWCA for twenty-five years and is co-founder of the Mayor's Health Task Force. She is fifty years old and describes her ethnicity as Hispanic/Latina.

Vilma was interviewed by Phillips Academy students Laura O. and Lily R. on May 7, 2020.

My name is Vilma Martínez-Dominguez. I was born on March 23, 1970. That makes me fifty; I recently turned fifty. I was actually born in New York, but as a baby was brought to the Caribbean, that's where I was raised. My mom was Puerto Rican, and my dad is Dominican and Puerto Rican. That's where I was raised back and forth. My hometown has become Lawrence. That's where

I have been most of my life. I've been in Lawrence twenty-six/ twenty-seven years. I am currently the Community Development Director for the City of Lawrence and I have been working in that role for almost the last three years. I am the mother of three adult children, married and living in the same place in North Lawrence since 2007. I am a grandma—that's one of my proudest moments. I have a five-year-old granddaughter. Most of my family, not all, is living here in Lawrence.

You co-founded the Mayor's Health Task Force. Could you tell me a little bit about your role and the initiatives that the task force empowered?

Substance abuse and then homelessness is our newest and I want to say most significant group. We have a large homeless population, unsheltered population, in our city, and now with Covid-19 it's been the focus of my work, creating two, actually three temporary shelters for people who are unsheltered, homeless and those who are housing insecure, which are those who are couch surfing, those who are living in double-up, triple-up housing, those who are renting rooms legally and illegally, those who are living in rooming houses. And so it has proven to be quite a challenge. But I'm really grateful because it's a lot of work, but through my lens of the Mayor's Health Task Force and my background in social justice, I have been able to frame a lot of the work that we do very differently. So I'm really excited about it.

What change do you hope to elicit in your community? In all these years of activism in the Lawrence community, what have been your driving goals?

I think we've done a lot together; we have been able to create change in so many ways. But it doesn't change the fact that we are a very challenged city. We are very resilient and we are very resourceful. But, with a city, with a gateway city particularly that's low-income, that's one of the most Latino cities in the Commonwealth, I want to say, in the region, where you have very low-income families, if you look at our unemployment rates, you'll say "Wow," they're very low. They're the lowest they've been in a while. But if you look at quality of life for people, we haven't gotten there. So, you have a lot of people who are working two or three jobs because they don't have a livable wage, right? And I think that impacts a lot your ability to prosper. I think that we need to pay attention. I know there's a lot of issues around quality of life that we need to address. Number one, and I think that it doesn't matter what conversation I'm having, the issue around housing and the high cost of housing. Most of our housing is rental and we have a lot of affordable housing but it's not enough. So, supply and demand issue here and it's gonna be one of the biggest things that we're dealing with and, again, with the quality of housing. So, we have very old housing and with that comes a lot of other contaminants, sometimes lead, and they pose public health and public safety concerns for many of our residents. And when you have people living—you know, ten people in one home, fifteen people in an apartment, and you actually have people renting rooms and there's not enough vacancy. Why do people stay here? Well, if you find yourself, your home, your community and you find everything you need here and they have created community here, you have your family, raising your family here. Nobody wants to leave what's good for you, right? And so, that makes it very difficult.

What happens usually, you see new immigrants continue to settle here, and so we are facing a lot of newcomers. I think it was probably six years ago when there were a lot of planning stakeholder groups and I was invited to be part of two stakeholder groups for two of the schools that were underperforming. As you know, our schools are under receivership still even though they are improving and there was, I believe it was 800 children entering the school system that year, brand new. And so you can imagine an under-resourced school system where you have probably many of the teachers that are here do not reflect us. Sometimes they don't understand the cultural component or don't have the cultural sensitivity to work with a population. And then you have a very densely populated school system. I mean, right now I think that the administration is looking to build about two schools just to fit the children we have here. And then you have Hurricane Maria. Hurricane Maria brought a lot of people here and I think that sort of compounds everything. The availability of good paying jobs, public safety. Some of it is perception, some of it is real.

We have made strides when it comes to public safety and decreasing crime, but you still see it. You see the issue around homelessness. It's the quality of life, once again. Small businesses, we have a lot of small businesses in our city. They're the backbone of our city but, you know, I worry a lot with the Covid-19. Even though there's a lot of resources available, many of our small businesses do not necessarily have access to those and I wonder what's going to happen. What kind of impact this is going to have moving forward. And so that's just to mention a few, but I think that a lot of these things we need to continue to work together. I don't think this is just a responsibility of our mayor or our administration, this is a civic responsibility. And I think that that's what made Lawrence the city that it is. Because we have a lot of partnerships, a lot of caring people. We have a lot of support; we have a lot of love for this city. I can't tell you how many people have come together with these three shelters. Right now, we have eighty people in one of our quarantine sites and we have seventy-two people in another one for the chronically homeless and we're about to open up one for isolation and recovery homeless who have no place to go to recover from this virus. And we have put this together in less than two months. It's just by the grace of God, by caring individuals, by people who are at the table who are saying, "how can I help." And I think that we're very strong, but we have a lot of work ahead of us. So, whoever is going to lead the city and continue to lead the city needs to understand these things.

You mentioned the coronavirus, I was going to get to that.

That's all we talk about these days.

Don't worry I'm going to get to that. I want to talk about the gas leaks in Lawrence (multiple gas explosions occurred in Andover, North Andover, and Lawrence on September 13, 2018). Can you talk a little bit about how you alter your goals to help the community?

There were different levels of impact from this gas leak and we're still feeling it today. A lot of small businesses in South Lawrence are feeling it. There's a lot of people who continue to be displaced because some of those homes were not able to open up again. We learned a lot about discrepancies in issues with housing and equality of housing as the inspection services and other people worked closely with Columbia Gas and to get the services back on. We experienced how even though there was a hotline, even though there were all these people helping and all these adjusters, that our community is very diverse and our community has very different needs and so not everybody could take full advantage of those resources that were there. I was there for the response, initially. The next three days we had to put together a shelter in no time. Again, with partnerships and the people that worked together in the city really made it happen. I remember the volumes of donations, I just cried. We stood in a corner, and we just cried because it was overwhelming to see the love for our city from afar. I mean there were people driving all the way from Vermont, from Maine just to come and help us out. But it took a long time and we're still dealing with the aftermath of that and so Covid now comes to compound that once again.

We also took advantage of National League of Cities, and they actually had a Mayor's Institute on Affordable Housing and Health. And it was the first time, I think, that we actually brought the mayor with us and some players came together to look at housing and health very differently. That's changing the conversations that are happening, which is needed before you can actually implement any kind of change moving forward. And so, everybody's now talking the same language and I think that's going to help us shape the future. Economic development right now, small businesses, many of them have struggled to get back on their feet. Our resources are great, but it's not great long term. These businesses need a different kind of support. We also need to think outside the box and we're really good at that because right now there's a lot of federal assistance from some of these businesses. But our businesses are run by families and so, if I have a sister maybe she's helping out in the business or maybe I'm paying her cash. I mean we never know. I may not be able to have access to the same resources that, you know, full formal businesses have. The much smaller mom and pop shops are hit the most.

I think that we also have a very young community and some- times ageism plays a part that we don't take the youth voices seriously. We need to tap into that. That's another way we have to say, okay look, this is a starting point, Covid is happening. Life is not going to be the same again, how do we incorporate the voices of everyone, particularly those who are most vul- nerable? You know, how to incorporate the grandmas and the grandpas into the conversation. And we've done that, actually we've done a little work with age friendly community, mean- ing we're exploring what systems and policies are in place. By 2035, in almost every city including Lawrence, the vast majority of people will be sixty-five and older, so how do we create a community that's gonna be welcoming and adapting to young and old? From birth to, you know, your elderly. We're looking at nine different domains and immigration is one of those domains, which is not usually the case in other communities, but we know that plays a role. So, what we have done is look at designations, for instance, housing choice, meaning that we have a commitment to create housing, at least 500 units. We're a green community that means that we have access to resources and opportunities to retrofit a lot of our buildings. I think that, looking in that sense, like really looking outside the box and being creative and looking at what other cities like us are doing is key for us to look forward and make changes. Business as usual cannot continue.

How has your life been altered by this pandemic?

So, this is my second month working from home, which is a blessing for me—but the isolation, remember I'm the oldest of six. Families are very important to me. Not being able to hug my granddaughter is killing me. And, to me, that's how I feel. Going to church and going to services and being part of that other community fills my cup and right now, I don't have those outlets. But I'm working to promote the resources that are available by going on the radio, speaking Spanish and talking to people about what's available for you, about where you can get food and what you can do to fill out your unemployment. That's how I'm sort of compensating some of that void that I have. It's focused my energy on that and then also the families that we're serving. These are families that have no place to go. These are families with children. These are families who are unemployed. These are families with a lot of needs. We have to have a shelter for these people with, you know, substance use, who are using substances and have chronic illnesses, and that's the way that I'm channel-ing my energy and staying connected.

But, it has impacted me a lot. I mean I have a twenty-one-year-old, that's my youngest, he's home from school. He's been home for a while now and that's a blessing for me. But it's also very difficult for people to be closed in, isolated all the time. I mean, our field trips, our weekly field trips are we go grocery shopping, or I go to the office to deal with contracts or I go to the shelters. That's the extent of the outlets that we have. So this is a moment where my faith is really being challenged. But it's also a moment in my life where I can reflect and sort of the fluff is gone and now you're looking at what is really important in life. So, what's really important in life is what you need to value. When we go back to the world, when this thing is over, I think it's gonna be a new day. I think we're gonna be thinking and acting very differently, because we may be dealing with this for a while and we're gonna be dealing with the aftermath for a while, but, it also makes me think at night and be grateful because I have a bed, I have a pillow, I have blankets, I have a heater, I have water, I have coffee in the morning, I have meals, I have my husband and my son here. We have Zoom. I talk to my daughter every day and my granddaughter and like wow, this is what's really important.

So, it has affected me. I'm a very social person, I'm a social butterfly. I love people. You put me anywhere, I'll talk to the wall. I'll talk to the flies. I mean, that's who I am and so right now that's very difficult. But, you know what, it's just one more challenge that we need to face. We have to remember where we've come from, what's important. Tap into those networks and that resiliency that makes us very special and just move forward. You can't sit and dwell, you gotta move forward. I don't know how this has impacted you, but being in four walls, this is my office every day from 8:30 a.m. to 8:30 p.m. or nine o'clock every day and that's my life right now. That's the other way that it's impacted me. Very long hours, all weekends, holidays, but you gotta do what's best for your community.

What do you hope to take from this experience after the pandemic subsides? What becomes normal after this?

It's uncertain. I think that we're seeing the numbers slow down a bit, both the number of people infected in our city and the people who are unfortunate or losing the battle to the virus. People's lives are changing right now. People are losing family, loved ones, and so I don't know what normal is. I don't think there'll be a normal. I think there'll be a new life: new opportunities, new lessons learned to bring to the work into our lives.

I hope that people reflect and understand. One of the things that is recommended, you know, the guidance is to wear your mask. Right now you can get a $300 fine if you don't wear your mask, but people are not getting fined. I mean, the point is, why not wear your mask so that we stop the spread of this virus? So, we can stop this isolation? And so you have people who are not following some of these things and it's resulting in a lot more people infected. There are times that you lose hope because you hope that everyone is in this together. So, it teaches you, at least to me that, yes, things will change but we still face a lot of different challenges and that's not going to go away. It's how we approach those challenges—it's the ideas, the creativity that we bring to the table moving forward. Right now, that's really gonna tell the story. But a new normal, I don't think there's gonna be a new normal. I think that even after the state of emergency is lifted and people say, okay, you can go back to your normal lives, I think people are going to be worried. I'm a hugger and a kisser and that's going to be very difficult. I'm very careful around that so I think those are some of the ways that are gonna change, but we are survivors, right? I've lived with a lot of difficulties in my life, we didn't have a perfect life, nobody does, but it's taught me to be strong and taught me to be resilient. I think that's the case for many people in this city. So, I think we'll figure it out, we'll figure it out.

***

Update

Since the onset of the pandemic, much has transpired in my life! For instance, while working as Community Development Director for the City of Lawrence and being part of the emergency response team that provided support and relief to families impacted by Covid-19, I also ran for office for the first time. My campaign efforts landed me in third place for the mayoral position, and although I did not move on to the general elections, I earned two national endorsements from organizations that advance women's representation in American politics: Emily's List and the Barbara Lee Foundation. I also received the endorsement of the Massachusetts Women's Political Caucus, and from many local leaders, such as former Lawrence Mayor Daniel Rivera, state representatives, existing and former senators, several small business owners, developers, and fellow activists. My political journey and my close to thirty years trajectory in the Lawrence community, promoting social justice and equity, captured the attention of many, and new doors of opportunity opened widely. Today, I am proud to serve as the Chief Operations Officer for the Greater Lawrence Community Action Council, Inc., one of twenty-three action council organizations that share the mission of promoting self-sufficiency and fighting poverty. Through my new role, I continue my life's work to help create opportunities for low-income residents in the Greater Lawrence and Merrimack Valley area— Vilma Martínez-Dominguez

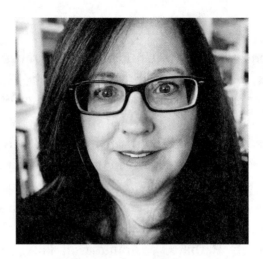

Felicia Sullivan

"A small group of people had formed a mutual aid group and I was part of that initial group that was formed. It is called LLAMA, if I can remember the acronyms [Lifting Lowellians: Assistance and Mutual Aid]. And through that mutual aid group, I was really struck by a lot of the urgent needs. It was trying to help people figure out how to manage when everything was closed down, especially manage getting food, getting medicine, dealing with school, dealing with the realities of being socially isolated . . . So, really trying to work with this very small group of people who are trying to figure out, how do we get food to people?"

Felicia Sullivan has been a resident of Lowell for over twenty years and is currently living with her partner. She is fifty-four years old, works as a researcher at a non-profit in Boston, and describes her ethnicity as Irish and Québécois. In this interview, Felicia talks about her privileges and how it has influenced her experiences during the pandemic. She also discusses the creation of LLAMA, a mutual aid group formed in Lowell to assist residents during the pandemic (For more information about LLAMA, please visit https://www.facebook. com/LowellMutualAid/).

Felicia was interviewed by Amir Cedeno on October 31, 2020.

So, the first question, how has your life changed during the pandemic?

Well, so in many ways, I am very fortunate. I have continued my employment and I work at a job that is very easy to do remotely, so that is the biggest change. Instead of commuting into Boston every day, I am working from home and have been working from home since mid-March of 2020.

I am pretty much a homebody person, so being at home is not a huge thing. Although, I will mention the curtailment of going out, at least to go out to dinner with friends or go to movies and those sorts of things. There were many months where we did not actually leave the apartment much other than once a week to just go get groceries.

We were also very fortunate early on, to have enough resources and not really feel any resource impacts on our lives, you know, like we certainly are very food secure, our housing is secure. Other than just the drag of being at home all the time and having to be extra cautious of our situation of coming in, those have been the major impacts.

Since things started to open up a little bit in the summer, I have started to go physically into work, once a week. My partner is out working now since mid-summer when things started to open up. So, other than some of the mental fatigue and drag, I mean most of our experience for the pandemic has been not hugely impactful. I think, the social structures around, sort of the politics and the uncertainty creates some anxiety. So, a lot of our impacts are in that mental/emotional realm of things. But my work has continued, in fact, it has gotten busier. I teach and do consulting on the side and those have continued, so we are very fortunate, our household is very fortunate in terms of the impacts.

Is there a particular story you would like to share about anything you experienced?

During the early days of the pandemic, in March, I have siblings in Georgia, so I had gone to visit them in mid-March and just when I came back is when everything really had closed down—almost that weekend after I came back, that mid-March weekend. I had started to do some work—even though I work in Boston, I am very involved with a bunch of different community-based organizations in Lowell—and a small group of people had formed a mutual aid group. I was part of that initial group that was formed.

It is called LLAMA, if I can remember the acronyms [Lifting Lowellians: Assistance and Mutual Aid]. And through that mutual aid group, I was really struck by a lot of the urgent needs. It was trying to help people figure out how to manage when everything was closed down, especially manage getting food, getting medicine, dealing with school, dealing with the realities of being socially isolated. So, with that group, these needs were very clear to me, especially for a group of folks who were very homebound and had either health conditions or life circumstances that could not allow them to leave their house. And then also, living kind of, materially on the edge, where food insecurity was a big thing. So, really trying to work with this very small group of people who are trying to figure out, how do we get food to people?

And at this time, in March and even into April and parts of May, the typical food pantries were not operating. They were not rising to the challenge of figuring out, how do we operate in a safe way? Many non-profits were really concerned about risks, legal risks, health risks, all these things. At the same time, there is this huge need of people who do not have food, have little kids or babies in their household or elderly people.

So, just trying to figure all of that out, like just a group of volunteers and neighbors, just trying to help each other out. I was really proud that there was a group of folks trying to put systems in place and come up with emergency responses. But I was also disappointed that our non-profit sector did not quickly rise to the challenge and was relying on just average everyday citizens to meet this huge demand. I was disappointed in our city government for not doing more, in terms of leading. I know they were concerned with trying to figure out, what if we have overruns of the hospital? What if we need to set up emergency medical stations? That sort of thing, but these folks were very desperate. I mean, I was part of the team, kind of receiving requests and figuring out where to direct them to and people were just in really dire circumstances, in terms of especially, food, and figuring out where they are going to get medication.

It became really overwhelming just as volunteers trying to figure this out. Even though I do not feel personally super impacted, I could see just by doing this little bit of volunteer work and helping out, just how stressed the system was and how dire some people's situations were. I was really proud of the average everyday Lowellians and people in our community, but I was really disappointed in our formal systems, our formal organizations, our formal government and their inability to act quickly and to respond to need and being very concerned about legal matters, and whether or not they were going to put themselves financially or legally at risk, which is how I inter-preted their hesitation to act. And this was compounded by our other governmental systems, not really responding well or supporting well. As things progressed, through the spring and into the summer, it started to get better because people started to adapt and started to respond in a more consistent way. But that inability for the system to respond to crisis in a quick way was really concerning to me and disappointing. I felt stressed out for all these families and individuals who just were stuck in their homes with little resources.

Yeah, so, I mean that is one of the most impactful stories for me and I think, then, followed by all of the racial tensions and the death of George Floyd, another instance of citizens just responding and saying, "No, this is not okay." For that I am very amazed at how average everyday people have been activated around things even in the fact that our systems have not been very good, in a lot of ways.

Did you protest?

I did, and you know, probably more like vigils locally and stuff, but it is also hard because people are trying to be socially distant. But also, I was just amazed at friends and family who have been trying to activate for a long time around these issues of racial injustice. All of a sudden, my brother, for instance, really seeing the injustice after many years of working and trying to get folks to see. In general, my networks are like me. They are educated, middle class people, for the most part living in segregated places and so I think they do not see a lot of the struggles that people have. So, I was just very amazed at how people all of a sudden were starting *en masse*, as a whole society, to see in a clearer way.

So, I think that is amplified by Covid, obviously. I think people being already on the edge emotionally and mentally and then just being stuck in their homes—maybe it has created a space for people to hear what communities of color have been saying for a long time. Maybe they just were able to hear it more or maybe their own lives are feeling impacted or stressed a bit. So, there is like a lot of not-so-great stuff about all of this but there are some really great moments of the larger society and individual people realizing things.

What's a typical day like for you now, as compared to before the pandemic?

Oh, the biggest thing for me is before the pandemic I used to spend a substantial amount of time commuting into my job, probably about anywhere from two to three hours a day driving into Boston or taking the train or whatever into Boston. So, now I am mostly in my home all day long. Most of my work has always been via computer. I am a social science researcher, so I am often working on projects where I am collecting data or analyzing data or working at my computer or organizing projects or anything like that. I was slated to do a bunch of site visits and field work to collect data, so some of that has changed; I am not traveling as much as I would have been.

So, my day mostly has me now in my condo, you know, working in my home office, on my computer. The type of work in general that I am doing has been similar. My home life is pretty similar other than, you know, my partner and I probably have seen a lot more of each other than we have ever seen each other, because we both work, have our social networks and are out and doing things.

I certainly am not visiting some of my local friends as much and I would have made a trip to visit my siblings again probably during the summer, but I did not. Both of them just happened to live in Georgia and so more being just stuck in my house, that is the major change. My work has not changed much other than I am in a lot more Zoom meetings and people seem to be meeting a lot more, which is exhausting. I have been teaching online for over a decade, so my online teaching has not shifted much at all, other than I might now have a few students who this is not their preferred mode of learning. Generally, I have students that this is their preferred mode of learning, so it is fine for them.

The biggest change has been not commuting into work: I like going into an office, I like seeing my work colleagues, I like being part of a social group at work, I like work culture and having people to talk to and seeing what is up. And so I have lost some of that sort of informal work culture that happens when you are in a place with people. My organization that I work for has tried to do that, like, create some of those opportunities in a more intentional way but it is hard, too, because people's workload has also increased a bit.

So, kind of minimal impacts in a lot of ways. I have not lost a job. My partner did lose income for a bit, but it started to pick up again in the summer, but . . . we do not have kids, we do not have elderly parents that we are worried about . . . I do feel a lot for parents who have little kids especially and are trying to manage school and manage home life. I was in meetings and deal with a lot of other academics and researchers, people and women who have very substantial professional lives and I just remember, especially during the spring being in meetings with women where all of a sudden, my gosh, they were just mentally frazzled, like, folks who normally are very cool and professional and you could just see that the whole home life and work balance had fallen apart for them, not from their own problems right, you know. The situation was just really impacting them a lot, I could see it in meetings and it definitely seemed gendered to me.

So, I do not have any of those stresses like, we have a cat. We have, you know, my major impacts are not that major in a lot of ways again. We are very fortunate; our household is very fortunate.

What do you think has been the most challenging?

For me, personally, the most challenging thing has just been the mental exhaustion, which I was not expecting. I was not expecting the mental and emotional exhaustion to the extent that it was, partly because I did not perceive huge changes in my life, just they are bad times and I am pretty super optimistic, but I tend to take things as they come and try to just deal with the reality of things. But certainly, as summer ended and kind of moving into fall, I, all of a sudden, just felt like a drag. It is probably compounded by extended periods, the changing season, our political environment, the uncertainty and anxiety that this is creating, just the length of all of this, of being mostly in my house for a long period of time. So, I think it just compounded. It was just shocking to me, I was not expecting to feel so dragged down, all of a sudden.

As far as your stress levels, how did it change during the pandemic?

I would say that most of my stress is almost always related to work. There was a point early on, like in March and April, people were trying to figure out what was happening, so there was actually in my work, a pause, like I had some time, I did some online learning and took advantage of that. And because work was trying to figure itself out, meetings got canceled, travel got canceled. But then as summer came and then into September and October, things started to speed up a lot. It is almost like people initially were like, "This is not normal, we need to take time, we need to realize we are in this situation, let us give people some space."

But at least in my work environment, that lasted for about maybe six to eight weeks and then it was like, boom! We are back to normal. And we have these deadlines. I work for a national nonprofit. We work with pretty high-profile funders and clients. There are a lot of deliverables we have that have to get done at a specific time, so that seemed to ramp up and they had been like, "No, these deadlines are coming." I had some major reports that had to get done and there was a lot and we move fast; we always move fast and so it just sped up very quickly and then we are meeting more. Like, we are meeting more, there is less time in the day to actually get things done. So, a lot of it had to do with work and how work was structured and then, having to work in this way that did not feel at all human to me, it just felt very like, let us get going, let us be fast, let us do all of this stuff.

Then, I also tend to take on extra things which I probably should not have done. So, I think, a lot of my stuff had to do with over commitments but also demands at work. Then, you know, I feel secure in my work but at the same time, we are in an environment where it is uncertain what is going to happen. It is a non-profit I work for, so is the funding going to be there?

Is there going to be work? Are there going to be layoffs? Is there going to be . . . ? You know, I am very confident that I am good, but you always have that in the back of your mind, like what if there is not funding? What if we do not have work? Will I be laid off?

And even so, my household is very fortunate; we have emergency savings, we are not anywhere on the edge, but it is always kind of in the back of your mind because we live in a country that does not provide a lot of social supports for people. So, I think it puts everybody on edge; if you are not independently wealthy, you are always going to feel a bit uneasy because there is no social safety net for people, so you feel like it is all on you if something happens. So that is mostly where my stresses come from. It is sort of like, feeling over committed, overworked. Luckily, my organization and especially my boss, is very good about hearing the stresses and taking them in and bringing them up the chain. Our leadership is pretty good about trying to manage all of this.

So, again, I am in a pretty fortunate place, but it still can be stressful and then you feel bad for being stressed out, when so many other people are so far worse off. Like, you know, my brother's income got cut over the summer. He is in a sales related position. My sister has school-age kids and trying to figure that out; I feel so bad for parents. In Lowell, just parents trying to manage, the school system is large, it is diverse, there is a lot of strain and . . . I feel so much for teachers and parents and kids and it seems like such a mess for people. I try to remember like, God! My situation could be so far worse; I could be in such a worse situation. So, I try to mitigate the stress that way, by just understanding there are so many other things that could be going on that are not going on for me. It helps.

Any other ways you cope with stress?

I watch a lot of Netflix and TV. [Laughter] I have probably

watched everything there is too, if you have seen it, I have probably seen it. I watched Netflix, Hulu, everything on cable, every movie, decent TV show, every Korean crime drama, every detective show from every country that is out there, like Broadchurch. It is just a way to kind of not think about things and just kind of edge out.

What are your favorite TV shows, if you can name a few?

Oh! I have got so many. What did I just finish watching? Well, I mean, one of my favorite series that just finished was on HBO, *Lovecraft Country,* which was really an amazing series. I do not know if you know it, but it is like sci-fi horror ghost stories, with a set of characters who all are African American, battling all sorts of things. So, it is just a really great series. I was watching a Korean detective series called *The Stranger,* which is sort of a quirky detective with his cop people that is pretty entertaining. What am I watching now? I start to lose track of everything because I have watched so much stuff. I am happy that the new season of *Star Trek Discovery* is on. I am happy that the new *Star Wars: The Mandalorian* series is back. So, I watch a wide range of things. I really like this comedy series *Schitt's Creek* which is like this family, this wealthy family that ended up in a motel after losing all their money and it is just a heartwarming series. So, I do not know, I watch a lot of stuff, I cannot pick a favorite, I just am watching everything.

Are there any positive aspects to your life during the pandemic, in particular?

Yeah, I mean I think, one of the nicest things is my brother early on started to host Zoom gatherings of our high school friends, which were quite fun—like people I had not talked to in a long time. My work has started to do some more conscious intentional social things, so this month, we are really celebrating Latin

heritage and so, one of my co-workers did a cooking demonstration of how to make this Mexican dish called *sopes*, which
are like basically fried corn, not quite pancakes but they are
flat. So, she did that as a cooking demonstration, and then she
and another colleague did some demonstrations of Mexican
folkloric dance. Then earlier this week, our People and Culture
Department hosted a Halloween Happy Hour. It is just some of
those things where people are a little more social and start to
build something, so I find some of those things are very positive.

Like I said earlier, I am very surprised at average everyday
people who step up, like the mutual aid group and then like folks
who have gotten out to protest. I am also amazed with how people are getting out to vote. Prior to my job I have now, I worked
for a civic engagement group for a long time that worked on
youth voting and so I am just amazed that people are out there,
voting. And in some places, standing hours in a line to vote, like
that to me is just, people are showing up. So, even if the systems
are not working, I feel like average everyday people are trying to
make things happen and do things. I think those are all positive
things. People are still trying to be creative and funny and yeah,
so that makes me feel pretty good.

How do you receive help when or if you needed it?

I have not needed a lot of help. I feel pretty fortunate and when I
do request help, it is usually from my partner or from my family
or my close friends. I got myself over committed in doing some
consulting work, so I reached out to one of my colleagues here in
Lowell, to help me out, to kind of take up that burden. I probably
rely on myself too much and probably should be asking for help
more than I do, but I am pretty well aware of resources that are
available to people and what is able to be done. And again, you
know, if I need recommendations, if I was trying to figure out
where there was Covid testing, knowing the right people to ask
for that.

So, I am pretty good, I have a good social support network. I have a good understanding of what resources are available and if I needed to go someplace, where I could go. I have been in Lowell a long time, so I know a lot of different organizations and groups and am pretty connected into things. I am a researcher, so I am able to figure out like, if I have a question, like quick. That is part of my personality, to find things and search things out and figure things out. So, yeah, internet, social network, you know, I have been working for a long time and I know people in various places around the country, so I am pretty good about figuring out where to go and stuff.

How do you feel about wearing masks?

Oh, I am pretty religious about it. I feel like we should do everything we can, to be very safe and I trust science, obviously. So, even early on I definitely wore masks. I was wearing one of those gator masks but then I read a study that said those are not as effective, so I stopped wearing that. And you know washing hands and hand sanitizer and even early on, when it was not clear how long this virus would stay on packages, we were trying to disinfect all of our packages when they came in. I think, we have stopped doing that, for sure. But definitely wearing masks, definitely washing hands, definitely trying to social distance as much as possible.

The places I find most difficult, sometimes, if I go to the supermarket at the wrong time, it can be more crowded than I want it to be. So, I try to go really early in the morning when there are not a lot of people there. When our office did open up, I was going in once a week. Our organization had very clear guidelines about how to be in the office, and the procedures to do, so our household really tries to stay on top of all that. I am not super old, but I am not young, so I am in a more "at risk" age group than someone younger than me. So I do think I treat it seriously. We have gone out to eat a few times, but we stay outside. It is mostly my partner and maybe one other friend, so yeah, I try to stay on top of the CDC guidelines and follow them as much as possible.

If you received a Covid test, how did that go?

I was not able to find a local Covid test for someone who does not have symptoms, but my partner gets a test twice a week and he is working at a university right now. So, I did not get a test, but I knew where I could get a test, like I knew if I had symptoms, there was a drive-up location. I belong to the community health center, so I am sure if I needed a test, I could go there and get one. Right now, I have not been in contact with someone, so I am not a priority person. I know Lawrence has been designated a high-risk place. I do not know why, since Lowell's a high-risk place, too, but there are no testing sites in Lowell for people without symptoms. But I know there are testing sites in Lawrence right now. And like Bedford and Fall River, like some of the places have testing sites that you can go to. And if we did have a free testing site, I would go and get one. In fact, that is what I was looking for the other day and then I realized like, Oh! It is not for folks in Lowell. It is for folks in these other communities.

Is there a particular reason as to why there are not that many tests?

I do not know why, I mean, Lowell certainly is a gateway city with an increasingly high risk. It is usually in that same list with Lawrence and Brockton and Fall River. And you can always tell when you look at a map, like, Oh! There are Lowell and Lawrence, whatever thing it is, they are always the color that is not the same color as everything around them. Like, Oh! There are those two red cities in the Merrimack Valley, Lowell and Lawrence. But yeah, for some reason Lowell did not have testing sites for people without symptoms. I do not know why, maybe, we did not have enough cases. Even though we have a rise in cases, maybe we just did not have enough. I do not know.

How have things been different for you, in terms of self-care and cleaning your house?

Well, I mean, we had a major household project. We had new flooring put in, so that was good. I have a bit of OCD with that sort of stuff, so that has been good self-care. For a while, I was walking every day, at least for two months, I was walking every day. Got out of that habit, but I have been doing meditation once a week and I have been trying to really be on top of that. I already like to eat a lot, so I just try to be on top of that. So, I have been trying to be a bit more attentive to that stuff, you know, when I was starting to feel a bit stressed out, trying to do a little more breathing. So, I feel like I have been doing better than normal because I am probably more aware that I need to do it.

What do you think the city of Lowell or the federal government should do, to keep residents safe and healthy during the pandemic?

Well, at least for local government, I feel like they have been good about messaging and have been good about working with the hospital and the public health folks. I think what the city government could have done better is, and maybe this might be the state government but certainly, the city government, could have been better at bringing the various nonprofit organizations and social service organizations together and really helping them coordinate, especially early on, things around food insecurity. Because at this point, like yes, there are the virus concerns, but there are these other concerns—mental health, food insecurity, housing. I think these things are going to start to really impact people even more than maybe the virus, like things where people's mental health deteriorates, where their housing slips away, where they do not have food, they do not have access to medicine. So, I feel the local government could do a little bit better at helping coordinate, what everyone is doing. I certainly feel like that is something they could be doing. I was happy Lowell put in place mask mandates and has been messaging Covid very well. I feel the federal government has fallen, has made things worse. I think, the federal government obviously could have helped states coordinate better, by a lot, understand where there were the high-risk areas, help with contact tracing, help with testing, help coordinate PPE, help states work together more so that every state is not trying to figure out its own policy, you know, not spread out so much disinformation about things where it becomes confusing, make it seem like Covid is not something to worry about, you know. Unfortunately, I feel like our current president [President Donald J. Trump] has not helped matters. On one level I thought like okay, when he contracted Covid, he might have been a bit more sensitive than after the fact, but it is almost like he doubled down on sort of, like it is no big deal.

Yeah.

So, I think he sowed a lot of misinformation and distrust of information, and it is very confusing to people to know what is what. I understand people who maybe live in rural areas or live in places where they do not see people getting sick or do not see the impacts, but when you live in urban areas, you see the impacts and you hear the impacts. The idea that folks could deny that is a problem, it is just amazing to me. So, certainly, the federal government could have done hugely better, by a lot.

Locally, I think we could have done better, too. As for the state, I do not know. I feel like the state has done pretty okay, although because I am connected to schools for part of my research, I do feel like schools and parents are very confused. So, I feel like at the state level, guidance around what schools should be doing like, they just reversed, they said, "Okay, if your city has been in the red for three weeks in a row, you need to close down and not have in-person classes." But then, two days later, they said, "No, you can meet in person." So, that creates a lot of confusion, partly because they are buckling the political pressure and so it is hard for people to know. And then you can say like, "Well, schools are closed but restaurants are open." Why can restaurants be open, but schools have to be closed? So, I feel there are a lot of those tensions between trying to be safe and trying to keep the economy going.

For political folks, it is hard for them. They are there because the voters put them in and so there is always this sort of public opinion they are trying to thread. So, I feel there is some of that sort of stuff that can be better, but if you trust science and you trust the information, the information is there for people to understand what you should be doing. The problem is, there has been an eroding of people's trust in science. Normally the Center for Disease Control (CDC) is someplace you should just trust what they are telling you, but the federal government has eroded the trust in that institution. So, infectious diseases are part of what they are doing, like that is their thing, that is what they provide guidance on and so not to trust what they say and not to trust that you wear a mask, things will be better. I was reading studies, clearly ventilation in buildings is a big factor of whether the virus will spread or not. So, people just do not trust the information. I get it but I do not know. I just do not understand it. I feel like the federal government definitely could have done better to boost our trust and not create confusion and havoc around what information to look at.

And respond earlier.

Yeah, absolutely responded earlier and unfortunately, it is the fault of our president and it is the fault of, primarily a senate, that has allowed the president to operate in a way that is not ethical. I understand why people will, you know, follow leaders and whatever. Yeah, but I think, had this been treated seriously when the first outbreaks were happening in Washington State and real efforts had been done to curtail it, I still think we would probably have had a problem but we probably would not be where we are at. And I understand the United States is a big place with a lot of people who want to do their own thing. Part of our national culture is to be individualistic but yeah, there is a way to message that stuff that would have not been government overreach, and it did not happen.

Is there anything else that you would like to add?

No, I am glad you and your class are doing this. And Lowell is a very diverse place and so, I think you can get almost every kind of story of the pandemic from Lowell. Maybe not a rural perspective, obviously, but there are a lot of different income levels, a lot of ethnic diversity, people in all kinds of life circumstances. So, I think it is a pretty good community. I find Lowell a very interesting place to be.

Well, thank you for your time.

Good luck, thank you.

***

Update

Since the Fall of 2020, very little has changed in terms of my work and day-to-day life. I have been able to travel a bit to see friends and family which has been a relief. The shift to remote-friendly work has made it possible for me to extend these visits so I can work from these locations and spend more time with people I care about. I am fortunate the health of my household has been free of severe illness including Covid-19. At the same time, I did hit a sort of wall of despair in March of 2021. Things had dragged on for too long. Still, I am also seeing some of the social life of pre-pandemic times starting to return. It is still very timid, however. My work has sped up as the nonprofit I work for has been well-positioned to take advantage of post-pandemic priorities. At the same time, I know many communities are still hurting and struggling to rebound—Felicia Sullivan

About the Editors

Susan Grabski has been Executive Director of the Lawrence History Center (LHC, founded as the Immigrant City Archives in 1978), since 2011. During her tenure, she has helped LHC create a more sustainable and effective organization on both a programmatic and financial level. In concert with the organization's development team, she works to secure operating and capital funding revenue. Susan acts as lead for educational programming, including academic symposiums and summer workshops. She has co-chaired planning committees for five community symposiums on topics of local, regional, and national significance and relevance to present day Lawrence community members. Topics have included the 1912 Bread & Roses Strike (2012), Post-WWII Immigration (2014), Urban Renewal (2016), Public Health (2018), and Public Safety (2021). Each have featured nationally known keynote speakers and attracted presenters and audience members from twenty-eight states and three foreign countries.

Susan earned her undergraduate degree in art history and English from UMass Lowell in 1992 and later earned her M.Ed. from the American International College in Springfield, Mass. She serves as a member of the Massachusetts State Historical Records Advisory Board, a Commissioner for the Essex National Heritage Area, and as Treasurer of the Board of the Friends of the Lawrence Heritage State Park. In June 2022, she co-authored a chapter entitled, "Lawrence, Massachusetts and the 1912 Bread and Roses Strike at Street Level: Interpretation Over Time" in the University of Illinois Press publication, *Where Are the Workers? Labor's Stories at Museums and Historic Sites*, a part of the Working Class in American History series. In 2013, she co-authored *Lawrence, Massachusetts and the 1912 Bread & Roses Strike*, with UMass Lowell Professor Robert Forrant, Arcadia Publishing, Images of America series.

Amita Kiley was raised in Lawrence and graduated from Northeastern University with a B.A. in American History in 2004. Her experience growing up in Lawrence fostered a love of the city and a strong sense of wanting to preserve its history. In 2001, as part of Northeastern's Co-operative Education program, she found herself working at the LHC as a preservation assistant. She continued her professional career after graduation at the archive. In 2015, she moved into her current role as collections manager and research coordinator. She works closely with LHC's director and local historians, coordinates and supervises volunteers, handles walk in visitors and school groups, and ensures that the hundreds of research requests LHC receives a year are answered in a timely and thorough manner. Amita is a member of the Organization of American Historians, Mass History Alliance, Society of American Archivists, New England Archivists, and the Strikers' Monument Committee of Lawrence, MA. Amita is a frequent speaker on all things Lawrence History Center and enjoys introducing others to their mission of collecting, preserving, sharing, and animating the history and heritage of Lawrence and its people.

Susan Thomson Tripathy was born in Rochester, N.Y., and grew up in the nearby town of Penfield. She first came to Massachusetts in the 1970's for her undergraduate degree in music at Mount Holyoke College, later returning to complete her doctorate in anthropology at Harvard University in 1989. Her dissertation fieldwork, supported by a Fulbright-Hays fellowship, was conducted in Jharkhand, India, and focused on the political and artistic history of Seraikella Chhau dance. In 1995, she began teaching cultural anthropology and sociology courses at Middlesex Community College's Lowell campus, and in 2011 joined the Department of Sociology at University of Massachusetts Lowell. At both institutions, Susan emphasized community engaged learning, frequently incorporating oral history interviews into her courses and student research projects. Examples of projects her UMass Lowell students have completed include facilitating a story-telling both for a Franco-American neighborhood festival; creating a film featuring interviews with people experiencing housing insecurity; and in collaboration with SayDaNar Community Development Center, compiling a book of stories describing the experiences of refugees from Burma as they left their homeland and arrived in Lowell (*Our Journey to the American Dream*, 2017, available at UMass Lowell's Southeast Asian Digital Archive).

In addition to her teaching, Susan authored a chapter in *Southeast Asian Refugees and Immigrants in the Mill City: Changing Families, Communities, Institutions—Thirty Years Afterward* (2007), and has co-authored several peer-reviewed articles on a variety of topics, ranging from case studies of a residential treatment center to analyses of how participatory action research may be used in engineering education to create a more supportive and inclusive learning environment for all students.

Remote Oral History Primer

By Mark Cutler, Lawrence History Center

What is oral history?

Oral history is the documentation of one's personal perspective in the greater context of a local, regional, national, or global story. Studying oral history testimonies, humans can gain insight into past events that "public records, statistical data, photographs, maps, letters, diaries, and other historical materials,"[1] alone, cannot reveal. Thus, oral history is a complement to traditional historical documentation, as it is a primary-source account of an event or events as one person lived them, and it can augment what other primary and secondary sources tell us about a time period. Oral history is a democratic process in that it gives equal importance to all people, whether they live in the public eye or are lesser known. As such, oral history affirms that every voice matters.

What is remote oral history?

Remote oral history achieves the same effect as traditional oral history, even if circumstances make in-person interaction impossible or inadvisable, such as the global Covid-19 pandemic that had people around the world sequestered in their homes and physically distancing themselves from the rest of society. There are many ways to execute an oral history interview remotely, including web-based conferencing applications like Zoom and Skype, tools that allow for podcast-quality recording of video and/or audio. Both Zoom and Skype allow for video interviewing as well as call-in access via a phone number. The recordings that these types of services capture can be saved on a local disk or cloud-based server and imported into editing software for trimming, composing, and curating archival-quality oral histories. Remote oral history allows people to make personal,

[1] https://www.baylor.edu/content/services/document.php/66420.pdf

human connections when they most need them and helps to highlight the lives of community members in a way that reflects the current reality.

What are limitations of remote oral history?

Remote oral history, at first, may seem impersonal and super-ficial. As highlighted above, however, during times of physi-cal distancing, this process may bring people closer together. Therefore, it is important for both the interviewer and the inter-viewee/narrator to recognize the limitations of remote oral his-tory and accept them as part of the adventure of documenting history in real time, across distance. Limitations may include audio and video delays, overlapping audio feeds, poor record-ing conditions, choppy video, "tinny" audio, and dropped calls due to narrow bandwidth or poor cellular signal, to name a few. You and the interviewee/narrator can mitigate these issues by following these recommendations, for starters:

- Ensure ahead of time that your technology works correctly and that you know how to use it.
- Solve any issues well in advance. Be on time for your call and even early if you are collaborating with a team that also is working remotely. This will allow you time to settle into the virtual space.
- Get rid of background distractions. Try clearing the space behind you, blurring the background, or using a green screen or virtual background.
- Use earbuds or headphones with a microphone to isolate yourself acoustically in the virtual space.
- If possible, situate yourself in a quiet place, free from back-ground noise and echoes, such as a bedroom, a closet, or a car, where sounds are absorbed by soft materials.
- The sounds your microphone picks up may interfere with the story being recorded. To avoid this, mute yourself when you are not speaking and remember to unmute yourself only to

follow up on something the interviewee/narrator has said. You also can use Zoom's advanced audio settings to suppress background sounds.

- Speak clearly and loudly and look into the camera when talking.
- Frame yourself in the camera centrally and visibly. Use balanced, controlled lighting to illuminate yourself fully from the front and reduce shadows and backlighting.
- When recording the interview, enlarge the interviewee's/narrator's picture and reduce or hide your own. The emphasis should be on the person telling their story—not you.
- Pay attention to the interviewee/narrator and give them your respect visibly and audibly.
- Mind your devices. Close all applications and turn off notifications that may make noise and/or distract you and the interviewee/narrator during the interview.
- Allow sufficient time for audio to transmit so that you and the interviewee/narrator do not interrupt one another.

For more information about how to collect remote oral histories: https://bit.ly/ROHPrimer